angry
Lonely
Tired

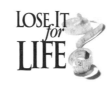

LOSE IT
for
LIFE

WORKBOOK

LOSE IT *for* LIFE WORKBOOK

Stephen Arterburn, M. Ed.

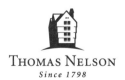

THOMAS NELSON
Since 1798

NASHVILLE   DALLAS   MEXICO CITY   RIO DE JANEIRO   BEIJING

Published in Nashville, Tennessee, by Thomas Nelson. Thomas Nelson is a trademark of Thomas Nelson, Inc.

Thomas Nelson, Inc. books may be purchased in bulk for educational, business, fund-raising, or sales promotional use. For information, please e-mail SpecialMarkets@ThomasNelson.com.

Material in the workbook is based on the book *Lose It for Life* by Stephen Arterburn and Linda Mintle, © 2004 by Thomas Nelson, Inc. Additional material and questions written by Len Woods.

Published in association with Alive Communications, 7680 Goddard St., Suite 200, Colorado Springs, CO 80920.

Unless otherwise indicated, Scripture quotations used in this book are from The Holy Bible, New International Version®. NIV®. Copyright © 1973, 1978, 1984, International Bible Society. Used by permission of Zondervan Bible Publishers.

Scripture quotations marked (THE MESSAGE) are taken from THE MESSAGE. Copyright © 1993, 1994, 1995, 1996, 2000, 2001, 2002. Used by permission of NavPress Publishing Group.

Scripture quotations marked (TLB) are taken from *The Living Bible,* copyright © 1971. Used by permission of Tyndale House Publishers, Inc, Wheaton, Illinois 60189. All rights reserved.

Scripture quotations marked (NKJV) are taken from *The Holy Bible,* New King James Version. Copyright ©1979, 1980, 1982 by Thomas Nelson, Inc. Used by permission. All rights reserved.

Scripture quotations marked (NLT) are taken from the *Holy Bible,* New Living Translation, copyright © 1996. Used by permission of Tyndale House Publishers, Inc, Wheaton, Illinois 60189. All rights reserved.

Scripture quotations marked (AMP) are taken from are taken from THE AMPLIFIED BIBLE. Copyright © 1954, 1958, 1962, 1964, 1965, 1987 by the Lockman Foundation. All rights reserved. Used by permission.

Produced with the assistance of The Livingstone Corporation (www.LivingstoneCorp.com). Project staff include David Veerman, Len Woods, Mary Horner Collins and Kirk Luttrell.

Cover Design: Brand Navigation, LLC (Bill Chiaravalle, Mark Mickel), www.brandnavigation.com
Cover Image: Steve Gardner, PixelWorks
Interior design by The Livingstone Corporation: Mark Wainwright and Kirk Luttrell

ISBN 10: 1-59145-275-9
ISBN 13: 978-1-59145-275-1

Contents

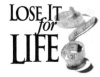

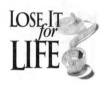

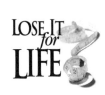

Part Three: A Lifelong Journey

Week 10: Community—the Connection Cornerstone

Week 11: Press On—Keeping It Off

Introduction

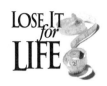

If you have read or are reading the book *Lose It for Life* by Steve Arterburn and Linda Mintle, you know that it is much more than a diet or a short-term fitness program. Lose It For Life (LIFL) is intended to be a way of life. That's why they say it's the "Total Solution—Spiritual, Emotional, Physical—for Permanent Weight Loss." It isn't about eating strange, tasteless foods or purchasing expensive exercise equipment. And the bottom-line goal isn't merely "to look better."

No, LIFL, is a holistic approach to health—aimed not only at your physical fitness but also your emotional, relational, mental, and spiritual well-being. Practically, speaking, LIFL is nothing less than an opportunity for long-term life change and permanent weight loss. It's about total transformation from the inside out.

Long before you stand on your bath scales shocked at the high numbers staring up at you, long before that new pair of pants suddenly won't fit, you need to understand that there are other, deeper issues swirling in your heart. The LIFL approach takes an unflinching and often fascinating look at these factors. Here is a summons to look honestly at *how* we interact with food and *why*. What is going on inside you when you make four trips to the refrigerator inside of fifteen minutes? Is food what you really need? Is your *stomach* really hungry? Or maybe is the true problem an empty or wounded *heart*? Are we at the mercy of such deeply ingrained habits? Can people truly change?

This *Lose It for Life Workbook* has been designed as a companion to the book, *Lose It for Life*. The two are designed to work together. The book offers you the information and tools you will need to understand what's lacking in your current approach to eating and how to begin the process of restoring balance in that area of your life. The *Workbook* gives you a tool for completing a wide variety of exercises and activities that are crucial to the process. It's an 11-week (5 days per week) program to help you reclaim the power to control your life in the area of food. To prepare for each week, you will be asked to read the appropriate chapter in the book. Then you should use the *Workbook* to help you wrestle with the issues raised in the book.

While not required for you to complete the program, the LIFL family of products has additional resources that you might find helpful, including an interactive *Journal Planner* and a *Day by Day Devotional*. There is also a teen version of the book *Lose It for Life*. Check out the ad in the back of this *Workbook*.

The *Workbook* has been developed to urge you to reflect more deeply. It will prod you to examine your thoughts and habits. It will ask you to remember past events—both pleasurable and painful. Mostly, it will push you to take all the facts and wise principles presented in the LIFL book and put them into practice. The *Workbook* is your private place to scribble notes, to jot questions, to record feelings and thoughts. The only rule? Be honest. Pretending never got anybody anywhere. Only the truth can set us free.

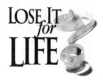

At times this *Workbook* will likely tick you off. You may feel like hurling it across the room. Please understand our goal isn't to elicit sharp anger or sadness. Rather, through pointed questions and practical exercises, we simply want to lead you to a deeper, richer understanding of *why* you do *what* you do; show you *how* you can shed bad habits for good and *how*, with the help of God and others, you can develop a whole new approach to life, to eating, to living healthy and free.

So read thoughtfully. Answer honestly. Work through the *Workbook* diligently. Pursue God desperately. Pursue connection with others relentlessly. And, lastly, expect realistically.

Do these things faithfully, and over the long haul, you *will* succeed. A healthier soul will lead to a healthier mindset. That will lead to healthier habits. That in turn, will result in a healthier body. Food will lose its powerful hold on you. You will shed unwanted pounds. Can you really do it? Absolutely! God has promised to help, and you have what it takes. Faith in a good and powerful God, together with personal commitment, is an unbeatable combination.

A final warning: If your goal is simply to drop 50 pounds as fast as possible, to get skinny so you'll look better in a bathing suit, LIFL is probably not what you're looking for. But if, at long last, you want to go beneath the surface—if you're finally ready to identify and grapple with all the underlying, unaddressed thoughts and feelings that have been driving your unhealthy eating and exercise habits—then we're ready to begin.

Buckle up. Let's get started. Let's begin to lose it for life.

Preparation: *Read the "Getting Started" introduction and chapter one of* Lose It for Life *before you begin the lessons for Week 1.*

DAY 1:
Losing It for Life

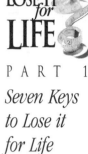

PART 1

Seven Keys to Lose it for Life

Despite all our diet books, health products, and billions of dollars spent on weight loss efforts, Americans are more overweight than ever. Obesity is a growing epidemic with 64.5 percent of American adults, or more than 120 million people, overweight or obese.[1]

Looking at Your *Life*

List the various diet plans you've tried over the course of your life.

Slim fast, phen, phen - La weight loss, diet for Heart patients, didn't eat.

How would you rank those diets, best to worst, in terms of long-term effectiveness?

L.A. Weight loss worked best
Heart diet - second
Starving - worst

What words or phrases describe your experiences with the assorted weight-loss programs and plans you listed above? (For example: "frustration," "the yo-yo syndrome," and so forth)

List the exercise regimens you've followed and/or the fitness equipment you've purchased in your attempts to control your weight. What were your favorite(s) and least favorite(s)?

tummy Roller thing
weights
tread mill
yoga mat - several workout DVD's

How do you feel—at the core of your soul—when you see an infomercial full of hard bodies hawking some new weight-loss or fitness system?

Some times Like there is hope.
some times Like they are full of bull.

LOSE IT for LIFE

PART 1

What words best describe your feelings as you begin this *Lose It for Life Workbook?*

This is to much writing.

Learning a New Way of *Life*

Losing weight isn't really the issue. We all know people with closets full of multi-sized clothing—testimony to the number of times they've lost and gained weight in their lifetime. Many of us are experts at weight loss. The real issue is, "Can we lose weight and keep it off?"

Why do you think our culture is so enamored with new diet fads and so susceptible to the promise of a quick, easy fix?

Self gratification, right then and right there

We don't want to promise hope and not deliver. We want you to be successful—to lose weight for life.

What feelings stir in you when you see a magazine headline that promises "Lose 10 pounds in one week" or when you see an ad for an exercise gizmo that promises "six-pack abs" in just three minutes a day, three days a week?

I believe it, and usally buy it.

Someone has observed, "It's not so hard to change; what's really difficult is *maintaining change.*" Do you agree? Why or why not? In what areas of your life have you experienced lasting change?

The authors assert: "There is no foolproof diet. Look around. For all our obsession with weight loss gimmicks, we continue to experience record rates of obesity. The truth is we have to change our lifestyles, learn to eat sensibly, and exercise. We know that doesn't sound exciting or terribly new, but it's a long-term strategy that works."

What do you think about this statement? Does it encourage or discourage you? Fill you with hope or dread? Why?

_____

_____

LOSE IT
for
LIFE

Losing It for *Life*

Whether you have long struggled with weight loss efforts or this is your first time trying to lose unwanted, unhealthy pounds, welcome. We want you to be successful, without feeling shame, guilt, pressure or condemnation. We know the weight-loss journey isn't easy. But we also know it is possible to shed excess weight and keep it off. You *can* lose weight for life.

Dream a little bit. How do you imagine your life would be different if you were able to reach and maintain your ideal weight?

_____

_____

_____

The authors state: "Lose It For Life is not about dieting. It's not about exercising, although exercise is a part of it. It does not promise a quick fix, a magical diet, or a thin body. Losing weight and keeping it off has more to do with changing how you think, feel and act at any given moment, rather than what you eat or whether you're in a regular exercise program."

Does this explanation surprise you? How does the LIFL approach seem different from other weight-loss plans you've attempted in the past?

_____

_____

The real issue isn't if we can lose weight; rather, can we lose weight sensibly and keep it off?

The LIFL plan speaks overtly and unashamedly about the central role that spiritual renewal and transformation play in one's long-term success. Spend a few minutes reflecting and writing about your own faith journey. How would you describe your own relationship with God? When did God become more than an idea or concept to you?

_____

_____

_____

3

LOSE IT for LIFE

PART 1

Lose It For Life is about creating a lifestyle of permanent weight management that emphasizes the whole you: your spirit, mind, body, and emotions.

In LIFL you will discover what essential ingredients are missing in your quest to be healthy in all aspects of your life. Look at the list below. Rank from 1–10 the current "health status" of the various components of your life (1 = "on life support" and 10 = "fit as a fiddle").

____ My general emotional condition

____ My family life

____ My friendships and connections with others

____ My work or school relationships

____ My optimism about the future

____ My ability to handle difficulties and setbacks

____ My overall view of things

Compose a short prayer that expresses your hopes as you begin this workbook. Tell God what is on your heart. Ask Him to do great things. Trust that He will.

_____

_____

_____

DAY 2:
The Culture of Eating

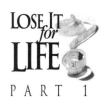

PART   1

Food is everywhere we look. Enticing ads fill the pages of magazines. Highway billboards loaded with pizzas and burgers grab our attention. Television commercials lure us to the refrigerator in search of late-night feel-good snacks. And if we really want to be tantalized, we can tune in to an entire television network dedicated to scrumptious food preparation and vicariously experience the ecstasy associated with eating it.

Looking at Your *Life*

If alien creatures visited and studied American culture for a week, what conclusions do you think they would they draw about us and food? About us and fitness?

_____

_____

To what degree do you order your days around food—lunch plans, dinner preparation, seeking out your next snack, etc.? Why do you think? Have you always been this way?

_____

_____

Would you say you live to eat or eat to live? Why?

_____

_____

_____

How often do you eat out? On average, in a typical week, how many "fast-food" meals do you grab and consume? How many "all-you-can-eat" buffets do you visit?

_____

_____

The same media that bombard us with around-the-clock temptations to consume fattening foods also broadcast a steady stream of images that convey the absolute necessity of being thin and fit. What is the wide-scale cultural impact of this mixed message? How does this food frenzy versus fashion/fitness craze play out in your own life?

_____

_____

_____

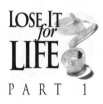

PART 1

Learning a New Way of *Life*

American culture is toxic in terms of eating. We are encouraged to pursue the pleasure of eating—whenever we feel like it. When it comes to food, we can never get enough; however, giving in to these hedonistic messages has serious fall out. We are fatter than ever. Our sedentary lifestyles combined with poor diet have led to an obesity epidemic.

Meanwhile, the cultural vilification of overweight people guarantees we will try anything to escape the stigma. The billion-dollar dieting industry plays us like a fine violin. When we aren't feeling momentarily defeated, we will embrace another gimmick and believe its claims even though those claims defy all logic. Our sensibilities are lost on the fact that if any of these dieting schemes actually worked, all weight-loss programs would go out of business.

Read Ecclesiastes 2. What did wise King Solomon conclude after his extensive experiment in pursuing pleasure as an end in itself? What is the lesson for us? Is food really able to satisfy the deep longings of our souls?

_____

_____

_____

Thanks to media images, any chance for a healthy body image is gone before puberty hits.

Jesus stated, "Therefore I tell you, do not worry about your life, what you will eat or drink; . . . is not life more important than food?" (Matthew 6:25). What do you think he meant?

_____

_____

_____

Most of us understand that you don't get something for nothing and that anything worth having requires effort. Why, then, do you think many people fall prey to "breakthrough" diet pills or natural supplements that promise miraculous results without a serious change in lifestyle? How susceptible are you to this kind of thinking?

_____

_____

_____

What are your current exercise habits? Have you always followed this regimen?

_____

_____

_____

The Bible makes it clear that God is the generous supplier of all the food we enjoy. For example:

> *"He makes grass grow for the cattle, and plants for man to cultivate—bringing forth food from the earth" (Psalm 104:14).*

> *"Give thanks to the LORD . . . who gives food to every creature" (Psalm 136:1, 25).*

> *"He has shown kindness by giving you rain from heaven and crops in their seasons; he provides you with plenty of food and fills your hearts with joy" (Acts 14:17).*

> *"God . . . richly provides us with everything for our enjoyment" (1 Timothy 6:17).*

Why does our focus so easily shift away from the great Giver of food to the good gift of food? How can we reverse this tendency?

_____

_____

_____

_____

Based on the verses cited above, is it wrong or sinful for us to enjoy a delicious dinner? Why?

_____

_____

_____

_____

In your opinion, where is the fine line between appreciating food and idolizing food? (Be specific)

_____

_____

_____

_____

LOSE IT *for* LIFE

PART 1

American culture has adopted an Eleventh Commandment —Thou shalt not be fat.

Losing It for *Life*

When we lose sight of the Giver of all pleasure, (food, taste, and eating included) and pursue pleasure as an end in itself, we carry a burden of excess, both physically and spiritually. We forget that our spiritual connection to a loving heavenly Father is where we find liberating truth, guidance for everyday living, and powerful help of the sort no advertiser or program could ever deliver. Lasting happiness will only be found in a right relationship with God and others.

LOSE IT for LIFE
PART 1

Our culture will not help you control your eating nor offer friendly support. In fact, it may oppose the very things that contribute to your losing weight for life.

Is this a new thought to you—that your physical health is tied intrinsically to your spiritual condition? Do you agree with this premise? Why or why not? Record your thoughts, observations, or objections.

_____

_____

_____

_____

In a few sentences, describe your own "willpower." How effective are you at setting and reaching goals? At summoning the strength to fight long-term battles?

_____

_____

_____

Many people who struggle with addictive or obsessive behaviors have found great help in the 12-step programs. One common feature of these programs is an admission of one's powerlessness to change and of one's need for outside help. How might such a confession help a person with a lifelong struggle against overeating?

_____

_____

God doesn't magically change us by "zapping" us. He doesn't routinely take away our desires for certain foods. Instantaneous, once-for-all life change is a pipe dream, not a reality. Given those facts, what are some realistic expectations for any weight-management plan you embark upon?

_____

_____

_____

DAY 3:
Control or Surrender?

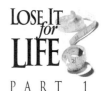

LOSE IT
for
LIFE

P A R T   1

Life is often difficult and uncertain. Just when we think we have things under control, something happens to remind us that control is elusive. The truth is we don't have control over much of anything. And until we come to terms with this reality, our lives will be full of anxiety, fear of the future, guilt over the past, and anger at others.

The key is surrender—surrender of our entire lives to God's higher perspective and power. Once you've made the decision to surrender all to Christ, true transformation begins. During the process, you'll meet (and need!) a "friend" who can really help. That friend is *grace.* Let's look closer at the struggle of surrender and this mysterious miracle called grace.

Looking at Your *Life*

Do you consider yourself a "control freak"? How much and in what specific ways do you try to orchestrate and direct the events and people in your life?

_____

_____

When have you felt the most out-of-control? What finally happened?

_____

_____

When it comes to weight loss/weight management, check off the following statements you find yourself saying (either internally or externally).

_____ "I need to stop eating so much. I need to just say no."
_____ "Quit being so lazy and exercise!"
_____ "As soon as _____, I will get my weight under control."
_____ "I can do this if I try harder."
_____ "I wish I had his/her willpower."
_____ "If I can just hit upon the right diet."

For most people, the word *surrender* brings to mind images of losing, giving up, being defeated and humiliated. But the key to victory in weight control is surrender. One key concept to grasp is grace.

How would you define *grace*? Give it a shot in the space below. (Note: Try to avoid religious lingo.)

_____

_____

_____

LOSE IT
for
LIFE

PART 1

*Grace is divine,
an undeserved
gift from God.
There is no
way to earn
God's affections
or coax Him
to love you.
He already
delights in
you.*

What is the opposite of grace? Or, what would a world be like that was devoid of grace? Describe it.

_____

_____

At what time in your life did someone—perhaps even God—treat you in an especially gracious manner? What happened?

_____

_____

Learning a New Way of *Life*

Through years of failed weight loss attempts, the road of self-effort and control has not taken us where we wanted to go. Proverbs 14:12 says, "Before every man there lies a wide and pleasant road that seems right but ends in death" (TLB). To stay on this road is to choose further heartache and destruction. Self-control and our various forms of self-help have failed us and must be abandoned.

What do you think the apostle Paul meant when he said, "When I am weak, then I am strong" (2 Corinthians 12:10)? How can acknowledged weakness lead to strength? How does this truth apply to those who are facing "the battle of the bulge"?

_____

_____

The Bible urges, "So humble yourselves under the mighty power of God, and in his good time he will honor you" (1 Peter 5:6 NLT). What does humbling ourselves before God look like in practical, every-day terms? What might this look like when dieting? Give some specific examples.

_____

_____

The authors say: "By acknowledging that God alone has the power to change the course of our lives, and that we are powerless to change it ourselves, we surrender to Him and begin the process of spiritual renewal. Only when we relinquish our control to God does He release His supernatural power in our lives."

What do you have to lose? (Other than stress and heartache and excess weight!) Why not acknowledge your weakness and invite God into the process? What is stopping you?

_____

_____

Grace may seem too good to be true. *There's gotta be a catch,* you may think. But God's grace is authentic, compassionate, and has the capacity to transform your life. Consider these Bible passages that speak of God's grace:

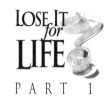

"[Jesus Christ] became flesh and made his dwelling among us. We have seen his glory, the glory of the One and Only, who came from the Father, full of grace and truth. . . . From the fullness of his grace we have all received one blessing after another" (John 1:14, 16).

"[God] has saved us and called us to a holy life—not because of anything we have done but because of his own purpose and grace" (2 Timothy 1:9).

What new insights do they shed on this subject of grace? According to John 1:14, who is the personification of grace?

_____

_____

Losing It for *Life*

Surrender is not passivity, nor is it resignation. It is an active, conscious turning towards God, reflecting our willingness to submit to His power and to share our truth with others. Surrender means:

- Admitting that God is all-powerful and releasing our struggles to Him.
- Refusing to escape into the old patterns, habits and attitudes that continue to distract us from destructive direction of our lives.
- No longer saying, "I can handle this myself."
- Humbling ourselves and submitting to God's way of doing things, even though we don't understand them.

Does the thought of surrendering in this manner excite you or terrify you? Why do you think?

_____

_____

Every wound and weakness is an invitation to God: "Please do for us what we cannot do for ourselves."

The authors compare and contrast a surrendered mindset with the person who is determined to remain in control:

Surrender	**Control**
God is the Master of the universe.	I can master all things.
God's perspective is higher than mine.	What I feel is all that is important.
My circumstances are part of God's eternal perspective.	If God is God, my circumstances must be changed now.
I must allow God's plans to open up before me.	My plans are all that matter. I demand immediate results.
I am not alone and will never be.	If there is a God, he is not a part of my life and I alone can change my reality.
I accept life, knowing that all things will work together for my good.	I blame God when life doesn't go the way I think it should go.

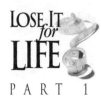

PART 1

Which column best describes the way you typically approach life?

_____

_____

In order to submit to God, we must trust that God has good things for us. Why is this kind of submission such a difficult thing for so many people?

_____

_____

Do you typically trust God or mistrust him? Why?

_____

_____

Grace understands the angst involved in doing what you hate—overeating, dieting, gaining momentary control, and overeating again—and says, "Hey, you can't do this on your own. There are healthy ways to eat but you won't make it with self-imposed rules. I am here to help you change your whole life not just your eating habits. You need me in your life." Will we trust in God's mercy and rely on His favor, even though it is totally undeserved? Will we trust in God's mercy and rely on His favor, even though it is totally undeserved?

Meditate on the jaw-dropping promise of Ephesians 1:8–9: "In him we have redemption through his blood, the forgiveness of sins, in accordance with the riches of God's grace that he lavished on us." The verb *lavished* means "to overflow, to have an excess or superabundance." No matter how much we've screwed up or failed, God's grace is *way* more than sufficient.

As we "lose it for life" remember that God's grace abounds in your life. He is for you, not against you.

The authors suggest a "prayer of surrender." If this prayer expresses the desire of your heart, take the time to say it now.

Dear Lord, I surrender my life to you. Open my eyes to the truth of who You are and what You desire to do in my life. Show me specific areas of my life that need to be surrendered to You. Help me to seek You with my whole heart. Lead me to those who will help me on this journey. Fill me with Your love and give me what I need to choose Your way and not mine. I trust You to love me, to take care of me, and to never leave me. Amen.

DAY 4:
What Works, What Doesn't

LOSE IT
for
LIFE

PART 1

You may be wondering, *Is the LIFL program any different than my past efforts to lose weight?* Perhaps you've yo-yo dieted, or lost a great deal of weight only to put it all back on with additional pounds. People approach weight loss with good intentions. In this lesson, let's explore the reasons some diets work and some don't.

Whenever you make a decision to change things about your life, there are costs to consider, and your heart cannot be divided.

Looking at Your *Life*

Based on your own experience with various diet programs, what are the ingredients of a good weight-loss plan? What are the marks of a diet that is destined to fail?

_____

_____

What is the most weight you've ever lost on a single diet? How long did that take?

_____

_____

If you gained the weight back, how quickly did you gain it? Why? Describe your experience. How did your weight gain affect you?

_____

_____

What has been the most significant *lasting* change in your life? To what do you attribute your long-term success?

_____

_____

_____

Learning a New Way of *Life*

Here are the most common reasons the average diet fails. Check the ones that you've encountered in your own experience.

_____ **Unrealistic expectations.** We often fantasize wildly about how different our lives will be when we reach our thin ideal. In dieting, if we begin with foolish assumptions, we are destined to become disillusioned and discouraged.

_____ **Overeating issues are not addressed.** Too many programs focus solely on how much we've lost rather than exploring the underlying issue of *why* we eat so much— especially when we're not physically hungry. A good diet plan will address these factors.

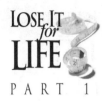

_____ **The diet is never personalized.** In the world of food and eating, one size does _not_ fit all. You have to develop eating habits that are balanced, provide proper nutrition, and that are tailored for you.

_____ **"Too much of a good thing."** Many think low-fat = guaranteed weight loss. Actually one can eat too much low-fat food and gain weight! Bottom line, we have to decrease amount and increase activity.

_____ **Medical factors ignored.** Certain medical conditions or prescriptions can contribute to weight gain. Before dieting, you need to know what is causing your weight gain.

_____ **Lack of support.** Research shows that social support helps sustain weight loss efforts and maintenance. Make sure you have supportive people to pray, encourage and be available when you need that extra push.

_____ **Superficial motives.** It is important that we are motivated by a desire for all-around _health_ rather than a mere longing for a thin appearance.

_____ **Inadequate exercise.** We cannot maintain weight loss unless we increase our physical movement.

_____ **Separating the soul and the body.** We are spiritual and physical creatures, comprised of body _and_ soul. A diet that does not take into account both aspects of our human nature is deficient.

_____ **Results were slow in coming.** Any lifestyle change takes time to incorporate. Remember slow and steady wins the race. Quick weight-loss methods usually fail long term.

LIFL involves no gimmicks, no quick fixes, no "melt away the pounds" creams or cookies that burn your metabolism. But there is a path to follow that will transform you. Healing, renewed thoughts, and meaningful connections will emerge if you commit to the process.

If a person wants only to be thin (and couldn't care less about being emotionally/spiritually whole), what are his or her quickest options to a skinny body? Why is this a less than desirable outcome?

_____

_____

_____

_____

Why is the support of others so important in an endeavor like LIFL?

_____

_____

_____

Read and ponder the story of Jesus and the rich young ruler in Matthew 19:16–24. What was the man's root problem? Materialism? A lack of spiritual desire? What do you think Jesus really wanted from this moral young man?

_____

_____

What does this story illustrate about counting the costs before making a decision, and the dangers of a divided heart?

_____

_____

The authors observe from this story: "Perhaps you are more comfortable with dieting than you even know. You try to be good—keep all the dieting commandments (Thou shalt eat only low-fat foods. Thou shalt have no chocolate before thee, etc,) and also wonder, 'What do I still lack?' Notice the specific answer Jesus gives. There is no question what is required—total surrender."

What do you think of this notion—that far more important than fat grams is *faith*, more significant that calories is one's commitment to Christ?

_____

_____

Is your heart fully God's? If you are holding back, why are you? What keeps you from giving yourself in total surrender to God?

_____

_____

Sometimes people eat for emotional reasons and because they are spiritually hungry. Weight loss must address all aspects of your life.

Losing It for *Life*

Let's identify the possible changes you may encounter if you lose weight for life. It is important to think about these possibilities up front. Some may apply to you; others will not. The last line is blank for you to fill in your own reasons. Take a moment and read through this abbreviated list (also found in the book). Check any and all that might apply to you.

In order to lose weight and keep it off, I might be changing . . .

- ❏ **A comfortable habit and way of life.** Eating is what I do when I am happy, comfortable, and feeling good. It's social and a way of life. Go to a movie without a bucket of popcorn? No way.
- ❏ **My best and most acceptable form of distraction.** For example, it's easier to think about the next meal, binge, or snack than the way my boss just treated me on the phone.

15

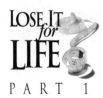

LOSE IT
for
LIFE

PART 1

❑ **A meaningful expression of love.** Food and love are closely associated. Cooking and eating high-calorie foods may be a way you give and receive love.

❑ **A way to satisfy needs.** Do I eat as a response to a felt need? Even though the food doesn't satisfy that need, I eat *as if* it does.

❑ **Protection from the sexual advances of others.** If I was raped or sexually abused when I was thin, I might believe that my weight has served as protection against further abuse. If I lose weight, will I feel more vulnerable? Am I ready and willing to face this?

❑ **A strategy to keep an intimate other at bay.** When I feel unattractive and don't like my body, I have an excuse to avoid intimacy (especially with my spouse). Am I ready to confront ALL the issues that come with building intimacy?

❑ **A cover-up for fears, including failure.** The reason I'm not married, the reason I lost my job, the reason I can't make friends…is because I'm fat. Could there be other reasons?

❑ **A way to control my life with false structure.** When I feel out of control, eating can be a way to structure my life.

❑ **A major coping mechanism for life's stresses.** A general pattern has developed. When I am stressed, I eat. Yes, STRESSED is DESSERTS spelled backwards!

❑ **My tried-and-true way to deal with boredom.** Boredom can be relieved by adding a little spice to life—with extra pasta, a little more sauce. When I open the refrigerator I find something interesting.

❑ **My best friend.** Food never lets me down. I can always depend on it being there and making me feel good for the moment.

❑ **My most dependable way to experience pleasure.** There is pleasure in eating, in taste, in texture. And hey, according to our culture, I deserve to feel pleasure (and lots of it!) whenever I want it.

❑ **The best or most acceptable numbing device used for emotional pain and anger.** Eating really works to distract me from emotional pain and anger. I don't have to think or feel—just eat.

❑ **Protection from rejection.** My layers of fat protect me from possible rejection. I don't have to date, ski, go to the beach, or assert myself—after all, I am fat.

❑ **Fantasy versus reality.** If I was thinner…ahhh, let me dream of the good life and fantasize about all my problems melting away with the fat. There's no need for reality to interfere.

❑ **A way of thinking that reinforces those feelings of not being good enough.** When I am overweight, I can continue to find reasons why people won't like me. They won't look beyond my weight to really get to know me. Without the weight, well…I don't want to think there could be other things about me they might not like.

❑ **Waiting for the future to avoid the NOW.** When I am down to a size 14, *then* I'll visit my relatives. When I fit into that dress, *then* I'll talk to men. The list for future action just grows with the weight gain.

❑ **Pretending I have no problems.** "Hey, I'm the life of the party, easygoing, and can get along with anyone. Everyone likes me." It's true. I never assert myself and instead pretend I don't have needs. I use food to cover hurtful feelings. My life is dedicated to helping others. It's selfish to think about me.

❑ Other:_____

LOSE IT
for
LIFE

P A R T   1

Ask yourself: If I embark on this LIFL program, will I be confronted with issues in my life I have worked hard to avoid? What issues?

_____

_____

Here are just some of the positive reasons listed in the book for deciding to "lose it for life." You will:

• Improve your health. As you gain a proper view of food and nutrition and become more active, you will lose excess pounds. Research shows that even losing a small amount of weight can bring physical benefit!

• Accept God's free gift of grace and become less judgmental as you are freed of your own guilt and shame.

• Become defined by who you are, not what you weigh.

• Gain an awareness of the difference between physical, emotional, and spiritual hunger and learn ways to satisfy all three.

• Find yourself more in tune with your body as you accept God's design for you as good.

• Take your negative thoughts captive, renew your mind, and think in more positive ways.

• Assume responsibility for your behavior and lose the victim position.

• Practice managing your emotions instead of allowing them to manage you. Emotions won't be frightening as you learn to confront them head-on and work through the pain.

• Make new and healthy connections with others—an important part of your recovery.

• Learn how to preserve spiritual gains and persevere to the finish.

Any lifestyle change takes time to incorporate. Remember, slow and steady wins the race.

Which of these positive benefits excites you most? Why?

_____

_____

Who are the people you can depend upon to surround you with support and encouragement in your LIFL endeavor?

_____

_____

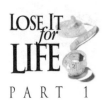

PART 1

DAY 5:
Ten Elements of Success

Congratulations! In a few minutes you will have completed the first week of lessons in the *Lose It for Life Workbook*. Hopefully, you are sensing a powerful new hope rising within. You are catching a glimpse that substantive change really *is* possible—not just another short-term spin on the old diet yo-yo, but real and lasting transformation, a brand new way of living.

Looking at Your *Life*

What are your biggest fears or concerns as you embark on this life-altering adventure?

_____

_____

Imagine being free from any and every sort of unhealthy preoccupation with food. Imagine being truly satisfied with smaller amounts of healthier foods. Imagine getting to the place that your body is toned and fit. Imagine enjoying dinners with friends and the taste of certain dishes without being obsessed. Imagine not lugging around all those excess pounds and feeling energetic. In the space below, write about some of your hopes and dreams.

_____

_____

Learning a New Way of *Life*

Romans 8:31 says that God is "for you." Spend a few minutes pondering that phrase. What does it do to your heart to realize that God is pulling for you, that He's in your corner, that He wants you to succeed?

_____

_____

A big part of the LIFL philosophy is recognizing that our beliefs determine our behaviors. When we engage in wrong behaviors, including unhealthy eating habits, it's because we've embraced wrong beliefs (see Romans 12:1–2). Therefore the deepest and surest way to change how we live is to change the way we think.

Can you begin to identify certain beliefs (about food, about dieting, about "thin-ness") or wrong ways of thinking (about yourself, about how to handle struggles) that need to be changed? Write your observations here:

_____

_____

Losing It for *Life*

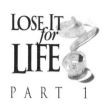

LOSE IT *for* **LIFE**

P A R T   1

If you truly desire to embark wholeheartedly on the LIFL plan, God will empower you to deal with the hurdles along the way. That is His promise. Through His Spirit, as you surrender to Him and accept His grace, He will transform you to His image. He is your help and source of strength. Invite Him to walk along side of you. His desire is to change your life—not just your body.

In the prior session (Day 4) we looked at the typical reasons most diet plans fail. This time, let's look at those factors that contribute to losing and keeping weight off long-term. These are the principles upon which the Lose It For Life system is based.

Ponder each statement below. In the space that follows, jot down your thoughts, questions or reactions.

1. You will set realistic expectations. This is how we lose weight, slowly and sensibly. (Other areas of your life may also require examination.) Develop goals but make them realistic and reachable.

_____

_____

2. You will eat at regular times in order to maximize your body's metabolism. The idea of "skipping meals" doesn't work. It sets us up to overeat, crave foods, and slows down our metabolism.

_____

_____

3. You will begin to exercise and move your body. In most cases, 30-60 minutes of exercise, five to seven days a week keeps the weight off.

The more active you are, the better.

_____

_____

4. You will monitor your progress. This means weighing on a regular basis and being aware of how your clothes fit. If you have a history of eating disorders, you may not want to weigh daily, but you will want to establish some accountability. In addition, medical monitoring may be necessary if you have health issues.

_____

_____

5. You will strive, by God's grace, for balance and moderation. This will become your mantra: "There are no forbidden foods." However, you have to exercise God-aided self-restraint for the sake of your health. It's the amount we eat and the reasons we eat it that matter most.

_____

_____

19

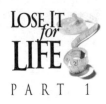

PART 1

Around the corner is true freedom— much more than weight loss! The decision is yours.

6. You must cut back on high glycemic foods (sugar and refined carbohydrates). For long-term success, feeling more energetic, and eating healthier, this is mandatory.

_____

_____

7. You will begin addressing emotional issues related to personal and interpersonal relationships. Filling emotional and relational needs with food doesn't work and isn't healthy.

_____

_____

8. You will cultivate a vibrant spiritual life. We are all in desperate need of a rich walk with God. We need to work actively to change how we think (Romans 12:1–2) so that our actions and habits also change.

_____

_____

9. You will enlist support. Research and experience are clear that we cannot find victory alone. We need to build community with people who will support and help us (and who we can support and help).

_____

_____

10. You will develop a more holistic focus. Lifelong weight control is an on-going process, that requires much more than a mere focus on body shape/size. Our emphasis must be on total emotional/spiritual/physical health.

_____

_____

Remember, surrender is the step that begins the process of losing it for life. Give up control. Trust God. Get to know Him better. Read what the Bible says about who He is, what He promises and what He will do in you and for you. "Taste and see that the LORD is good. Blessed is the man [and woman] who takes refuge in him" (Psalm 34:8).

Preparation: Read chapter two of Lose It for Life *before you begin the lessons for Week 2.*

DAY 1:
The Matrix . . . or Reality?

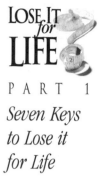

LOSE IT *for* LIFE

PART 1

Seven Keys to Lose it for Life

The film *The Matrix* tells the story of a computer hacker named Neo who lives a rather ordinary life in what he thinks is the year 1999. Then he meets a man named Morpheus, who explains to Neo that his reality is false. It is actually 200 years later, artificial intelligence runs the world, and all humans are trapped in a complex computer "matrix" in which they are used for fuel to run the machines. Morpheus gives Neo a life-altering choice. He can go on living in his false world or he can *take the red pill.* Once he swallows the red pill, he'll see life as it really is!

LIFL confronts you with a similar life-altering choice. Do you want to continue to live in the false world of dieting, where emotional pain is numbed, health risks are ignored, and false promises are made? Or do you want to "take the red pill" and see the reality of a world in which food and eating don't dominate your life or take over? If you take the challenge, you will have to face things you have avoided, deal with relationship difficulties, and make changes in your lifestyle.

Looking at Your *Life*

How we spend our hours is how we spend our days, and how we spend our days is how we spend our lives. All of us are headed in a certain trajectory; unless we do something to alter our direction, we will end up where we are headed.

How are you spending your days? Where are you headed?

_____

_____

If you don't change some things about how you think about and deal with food, about how you take care (or don't take care) of your body and soul, where do you think you will you end up? (Try to project 10, 20, or 30 years into the future.)

_____

_____

Would the people who know you best and love you most say that you are a wide-eyed realist or someone who easily falls prey to deceptive ideas? Would they say you more readily take responsibility for your life situation or that you are prone to make excuses, justify, rationalize, and blame others?

_____

_____

Dostoevsky's novel *The Brothers Karamazov* is a classic. One of the main characters observed, "The important thing is to stop lying to yourself. A man who lies to himself, and believes his lies, becomes unable to recognize the truth, either in himself or anyone else, and he ends up losing respect for him-

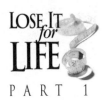

P A R T   1

*We can
facilitate
change. . . .
But you will
have to make
some hard
decisions and
re-evaluate
your motiva-
tions for
wanting to
lose weight.*

self as well as others. When he has no respect for anyone, he can no longer love and . . . behaves in the end like an animal, in satisfying his vices."

When it comes to your relationship with food, are you lying to yourself? (Be honest!)

_____

_____

Learning a New Way of *Life*

In order to lose weight for life, we have to face reality or we end up lying to ourselves and to others. We must ask (and answer) tough, uncomfortable questions such as:

- What is *my* part in gaining weight?
- How do I respond to difficulty?
- What unmet needs do I have that I try to meet through food?
- When life gets tough, do I get going or start eating?
- Am I hung up on *why* my life feels so out of control?
- Am I disconnected from others?
- Am I in denial?

What are your "first blush" reactions to these probing queries?

_____

_____

Read John 16:33 in your Bible. "In this world you will have trouble," Jesus said. Difficulty and suffering will be part of life. How does that reality make you feel?

_____

_____

In the same breath, Jesus offered hope. "Take heart! I have overcome the world." During His life on earth, He overcame temptation from Satan. Through His death on the cross and the power of His resurrection, He destroyed the power of sin and death. Now He is able to offer otherworldly peace and freedom—a whole new way of living.

When it comes to food and weight and dieting, are you more often "at war" within, or flooded with God's peace? Why?

_____

_____

_____

22

When is the last time you felt truly at peace, relaxed to the depths of your soul? What were the circumstances? What would it be like to experience a whole life of such "rest"?

_____

_____

As the perfect Son of God, Jesus is incapable of lying. He can only tell the truth. What does John 14:6 reveal about the character of Christ?

_____

_____

The psalmist prayed: "Lord, you have examined my heart and know everything about me" (Psalm 139:1 NLT). How can this fact free us up to be honest with God, others, and ourselves?

_____

_____

Losing It for *Life*

We take steps toward true freedom and true peace when we soberly and realistically decide to "take the red pill." We choose to give up our false and foolish ways of thinking and living, and accept certain truths:

- My overweight body is a symptom of an underdeveloped soul.
- No one else caused my problem and no one else is going to fix it for me.
- When I decide to change, it is going to be painful.
- No one can walk through that pain but me, and I *must* walk through it.

Record your true thoughts about these statements:

_____

_____

In the LIFL book, the authors state: "All of us struggle with blind spots in our lives, and to some degree live in denial and self-deception. Rather than confront our area of struggle and pain, we often point to others and focus on them, or find ways to distract and anesthetize ourselves."

Do you agree? Why or why not?

_____

_____

Acceptance is being willing to see, to lift the curtain of denial and look unblinkingly at the "big lie" of your life. Breaking through denial means being aware of your struggle and pain and consciously confronting the behaviors and patterns that have detoured you from God's best.

"You will know the truth, and the truth will set you free" (John 8:32).

23

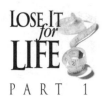

PART 1

With God's help, remove the blinders of deception and denial. Begin to see yourself as you really are. Then see God as He is: patient and loving.

Take a moment and rigorously examine your heart. Ask God for the courage to be brutally honest. How have you avoided reality? How many (if any) of these truth-avoiding "symptoms" are a regular part of your life? Check all that apply.

____ I avoid honest prayer.

____ I avoid times of silence.

____ I avoid discussions that focus on my life situation.

____ I avoid honest conversations that touch on sensitive or painful areas of my life.

____ I avoid people who can (and would) speak into my life and encourage me on the journey.

____ I minimize or rationalize my behavior and its affect on others.

____ I find myself constantly criticizing or pointing the finger at others—either outwardly or inwardly.

____ I am confused as to why others react the way they do to me, and what I say or do.

____ I catch myself lying repeatedly—or stretching and twisting the truth.

Here's how you'll have to change if you want to leave behind a life of delusion and excuse-making. Here are the positive signs that will mark your life:

- You will focus on what *you* can do to change rather than on what you want others to do to make you feel better.
- You will humble yourself in order to see and confront who you really are.
- You will look hard for what really causes the conflicts you experience.
- You will honestly face your past, pain and failures head on.
- You will stop blaming others for your difficulties.
- You will actively seek, receive and apply God's wisdom to your situation.
- You will look at what you've done in the light of God's mercy and grace—not judgment or condemnation.
- You will accept that you are unable to change without God's help.
- You will name your character defects and mistakes rather than deny them.

What's your gut-level reaction to this list? What hopes or fears are stirred in you as you contemplate it?

_____

_____

By being humble, courageous, and honest, we can move out of the past and into the reality of the present where God can teach us to resolve our problems rather than reproduce them in family and close friends. Are you ready to take the red pill?

DAY 2:
Letting Go of Excuses

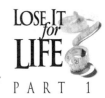

LOSE IT
for
LIFE

P A R T   1

Are you ready to be completely honest with yourself and others and stop making excuses for why your life is the way it is?

Looking at Your *Life*

What are your five best qualities?

_____

_____

What are your three worst habits?

_____

_____

How about "making excuses" for your eating/exercise habits? Are you guilty? On a scale of 1–10, with 1 being "I'm afraid I do it all the time!" and 10 being "I *never* make excuses!" how would you rank yourself?

_____

_____

The LIFL authors give the following example in the book:

It's late at night. You are watching TV and you start thinking about ice cream because you've just seen a tantalizing commercial. Anxiety begins to mount as you try to decide if you should eat the ice cream sitting in your freezer…or say no. You aren't thinking about the fact that you are *not* hungry. The ice cream just looks so good—it would be a terrific treat right now…and it's calling to you from the freezer…and you've had a long and exhausting day. All of these are excuses that hide the truth: *You are not hungry.* But the excuses come so easily, so smoothly, it has become your habit to just ignore the truth when it comes to overeating. Excuses take the focus off of the long-term consequences.

Certainly you don't want to think about the long-term effects of overeating right now. And the longer you postpone eating the ice cream, the greater your anxiety becomes. "Should I eat or shouldn't I?" Eventually you become so uncomfortable over this dilemma that you get up, walk to the kitchen, and serve yourself a scoop of ice cream.

Then you think, *There isn't that much ice cream left in the carton. I'll finish it off and won't buy anymore. I'll start dieting tomorrow when it's all gone.* As you begin to overeat, the

25

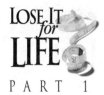

PART 1

*Excuses are
simply ways
we lessen
momentary
anxiety so we
can overeat.*

momentary anxiety disappears. The ice cream tastes great, or at least you think it did—you ate it so fast, you really didn't taste it. Now it's late, and now you are really tired. Feeling uncomfortably full, you go to bed.

When do you most often catch yourself in similar situations as the ice cream example?

_____

_____

_____

Learning a New Way of *Life*

Giving in to strong, momentary urges (in order to ward off anxious feelings) is a dangerous habit. By refusing to think about long- term consequences, we become pawns or puppets in the hands of advertisers. Think about it—immediate gratification is the strong, underlying message of every ad or commercial. The whole marketing industry is designed to persuade us to think and act impulsively. If we're ever going to find true freedom and peace and victory, we must learn a new way of thinking and living.

Are you a short-term thinker or a long-term thinker? Why do you say that? What would your friends and family say?

_____

_____

_____

Circle the statement in either column that best describes how you usually react.

I react impulsively.	**I respond thoughtfully.**
1. $100! Let's go to the mall!	$100! Maybe I should save this?
2. I do things spur of the moment.	I like to plan things out in advance.
3. I'm blunt. I say what's on my mind.	I'm tactful. I fret over how to say hard things.
4. I don't know what I'm doing next week.	I have a life plan or personal mission statement.
5. I buy my Christmas gifts at the last minute.	I Christmas shop far in advance.
6. Retirement? 401K? IRA? Ha!	I just got back from an appt. with my financial planner.
7. My kids? Hmmm. I guess they're okay.	I'm deeply concerned about my kids' futures.
8. Sounds good to me! Let's do it.	How could this decision affect others?
9. What would feel good now?	What is God calling me to be and do?
10. You only go around once in life.	One day I will stand before God.

How common is it for you to stop (before eating) and ask questions such as these?

- How will I feel after I eat this?
- How will I feel in thirty minutes?
- How will I feel about this tomorrow morning?
- Will I beat myself up over this?

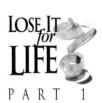

PART 1

_____

_____

_____

If you're not in that habit, what would it take for you to develop this habit—thinking through the ramifications of your decisions?

_____

_____

Read Galatians 5:22–23. This passage depicts the character qualities of a person who is surrendered to God's Spirit and living under His control. Notice the last "fruit of the Spirit" listed. What does this suggest to you? What hope does this give in the whole weight-loss/weight-control battle?

_____

_____

_____

Fruit always comes from a seed. Interestingly, Jesus spoke of the Word of God as being like seed (Luke 8:1–15). What are the implications of this? What role does the Bible play in learning to lose it for life?

_____

_____

How—realistically and practically—do we plant the seed of God's Word deeply in our lives so that it bears fruit over time?

_____

_____

The original temptation to sin involved food (Genesis 3), as did Christ's temptation in the wilderness. Read Luke 4:1–13. How did Jesus fight the lure of immediate gratification?

_____

_____

_____

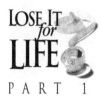

PART 1

Here are some practical, tried and true suggestions for battling the anxious temptations to overeat (or to eat when you're not really physically hungry):

- Tell yourself, "It's normal to feel anxious when making a change. This feeling will pass shortly."
- Breathe deeply and relax your body. Usually the urge subsides within 20 minutes or so.
- Distract yourself with something else. Turn off the TV, pull out a book, go to the bathroom (people tend not to eat in the bathroom), take a walk, chew some sugar-free gum, or go to bed. Don't stare at the refrigerator and try to exercise will power.
- Try to avoid tempting situations all together. If you are realizing that late night TV viewing is a trigger for you to overeat, don't watch late night TV! Do something different— play a game, read a good book, pray for your family, work on a Bible study, and so forth.
- If you do decide to eat, eat a piece of fruit, chewing it slowly. Or go ahead and take *one* small scoop of ice cream and no more. Eat it slowly and enjoy every bite. You won't gain a pound from one small scoop, but eating the entire carton will do some damage.

Which of these suggestions do you think will work best for you? Why?

_____

_____

Jesus' defense against succumbing to immediate gratification was to quote God's Word to His enemy. That's our model for overcoming.

Losing It for *Life*

A big part of the LIFL approach is taking responsibility. We stop blaming others for our situation. We surrender to God, trusting Him to do what we cannot do, and we take responsibility for doing all that we can. Responsibility also means confronting old wounds that can trigger our overeating. We could fill volumes with the stories of people who have used overeating as a way of numbing emotional hurts. Perhaps you, too, have spent your life anesthetizing your emotions with food rather than addressing your disappointments and grief. LIFL wants to provide you with the truth and encouragement to face your pain and grieve your losses, so that you find deep healing.

There is much psychological talk about our "victim" culture. What does this mean? Why are so many so quick to take on the role of victim and live a life of victimization?

_____

_____

King David wrote, "It was good for me to be afflicted so that I might learn your decrees" (Psalm 119:71). How can affliction and pain end up serving God's good purposes for our lives?

_____

_____

The authors state: "Avoiding pain and problems is a natural human response. Most people feel they have 'suffered enough' and have no desire to feel overwhelmed by sorrowful emotions. But grief is a necessary process in life. Grief over our failures and losses connects us to God's grace. Saint Augustine affirmed this when he said, 'In my deepest wound I saw your glory and it dazzled me.'"

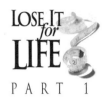

How do you respond to that thought? Is this a new perspective for you?

_____

_____

It would be easy to use your past pain as a lifelong excuse for not changing (but you'd miss God's best). Many people choose to live this way. It would also be easy to blame others for everything that has gone wrong in your life. Accepting responsibility is a bold step, and a better way.

Are you willing to . . .

- ❏ Face your problems rather than run from them?
- ❏ Take the time now to finally grieve your losses?
- ❏ Believe Jesus' words, "Blessed are those who mourn for they will be comforted"?
- ❏ Stop playing the role of victim?
- ❏ Bear the full responsibility of your own misconduct
- ❏ Reach out to Christ, who is fully capable of understanding your emotional pain because He suffered abuse and rejection Himself?
- ❏ Look beyond your loss to God's deeper purposes?
- ❏ Accept the hope that God's plans for you are good and loving?
- ❏ Refuse to allow anything from your past to be an excuse for lack of growth or character development?

If you checked any boxes, you have taken a wise and courageous step! We applaud your brave heart. With God's truth, God's power, God's indwelling Spirit, and God's people, you can lose it for life—by appropriating fully the new life that Christ gives!

The book offers a prayer for accepting responsibility. If you wish, pray it silently right now.

Dear Lord,
I realize that you have given me life and my life is my responsibility. I know You want my life to be fruitful, but sin and tragedy has infected my life—both by my hand and the hand of others. Help me to accept responsibility to remove these weeds that have been sown in me. Lord, I confess that sometimes I blame others for my own disobedience to You. I now accept responsibility for these things. Please forgive me and fully restore the relationships between us. Amen.

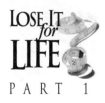

DAY 3:
New Motives and Methods!

Once you have decided to give up a lifestyle of making excuses, and after you have prayed through your acceptance and responsibility, then it's time to examine your motivation for wanting to lose weight.

Looking at Your *Life*

If you had a magic wand and could wave it over your life, what three big changes would you most like to see and why?

_____

_____

_____

_____

Research tells us that people become more successful at long-term weight loss when their motivation is to become healthier not thinner.

Our emotions are the warning lights on the dashboard of our lives. When we find ourselves flashing with a strong emotion—fear, anger, worry, sadness—it's time to "pull over" so to speak, and "look under the hood" at what's really going on inside us. Does the idea of self-examination trouble you or excite you? Why?

_____

_____

_____

_____

_____

Be honest—which of the following options might you choose? Why would you choose that?

- Living another *thirty* years, while enjoying an absolutely flawless physique—a body off the cover of some magazine.
- Living another *fifty* years, in a reasonably fit and healthy body—though not necessarily a body that would cause people to stop and stare in envy.

_____

_____

_____

_____

_____

Learning a New Way of *Life*

As you learn more about making good food choices and self-care, your focus should be on becoming a healthier, not thinner you. This change in attitude and motivation is essential.

If one's goal is merely to look more attractive, rank the following ways to do that, from 1–10 (1=most effective; 10=least effective):

_____ liposuction and other forms of plastic surgery

_____ gastric bypass surgery

_____ vegetarian diet

_____ low-fat diet

_____ low-carb diet

_____ aerobics classes

_____ new wardrobe

_____ cosmetic dental surgery

_____ tanning booth sessions

_____ weight/strength-training

LOSE IT
for
LIFE

PART 1

"I am the LORD, the God of all mankind. Is anything too hard for me?" (Jeremiah 32:27).

If one's goal is to become an overall healthier, happier person, what activities might need to be added to the above list and why?

Healthy Habit or Practice	Why & How This Contributes to Overall Health

Read 1 Timothy 4:7–8. What does this passage suggest is important in achieving overall health?

_____

_____

_____

In Philippians 4:13, the apostle Paul exclaims, "I can do everything through him who gives me strength." What is the significance of this statement to those who are opting for the long-term view of life-long weight loss/management?

_____

_____

31

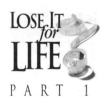

PART 1

Studies also show that people who record what they eat lose more weight and keep it off compared to those who don't.[1]

Losing It for *Life*

Perhaps you are frustrated because it seems as though you've been dieting forever and haven't lost a pound. We know the drill!

In the LIFL book, Dr. Linda tells of her college "cottage cheese diet" which helped her *gain* fifteen pounds her freshman year. She reports how she skipped breakfast everyday (food or sleep was my option), ate cottage cheese and fruit for lunch, and ate a regular dinner. Staring daily at her little bowl of white mealy curd lunch, she believed she was making the ultimate sacrifice to lose weight. She ate it religiously and thought the pounds would fall off.

What she "forgot" to add to the equation were her nightly visits to the dormitory snack machines. In addition to her 7 A.M. to 7 P.M. dietary discipline, Dr. Linda was also ingesting late night fruit pies and cinnamon buns and Doritos ® and chips and chocolate. Add up all those extra "study snack" calories that didn't "count" because they weren't part of her "healthy" meals, and it's no wonder she didn't lose weight.

What are your snack habits?

_____

_____

_____

_____

When do you find yourself most susceptible to nibbling and grazing?

_____

_____

_____

_____

Research shows that very few people have metabolic disorders or genetic factors that cause overweight. The truth is that most people grossly underestimate what they eat in a day and they exercise far less than they think.[2] It's not that people intentionally lie about what they eat. They just forget all those random moments in the day when they grab a handful of chocolates or taste a few spoonfuls of chili while preparing dinner. A little here, a little there adds up.

Get a small blank tablet that you can carry with you. Begin right now writing down everything you eat in a day for a week or two. This may sound tedious, but it will provide you with a greater awareness of what you are eating. The food journal will also pinpoint eating patterns—when you eat, how much, how often, what you eat, etc. This information will later be used to make changes.

Find a companion who will do this with you. Having a partner to remind you and encourage you is a great way to develop this new, important habit. Use the following format to help monitor your progress.

Food Journal

Name: Jane Doe   **Day:** Wednesday, May 18

When I ate?	Where?	What I ate?	How much?	Was I Hungry?
Breakfast (8:00 a.m.)	Kitchen table	Jelly donuts	3	Yes
		Coffee	3 cups, 3 Tbls cream, 2 Tbls sugar	
		Orange Juice	8 oz glass	Yes
Snack (10:00 a.m.)	Desk at work	Pop Tart	2	Yes

After you have set up your food journal, commit this exercise to God with this prayer:

Father,
I have begun this new adventure that I hope and pray will become a new way of life. I do not want to be controlled by food or by unhealthy emotions. Give me the grace to lean on you at all times. Help me change my mindset so that I am motivated by a deep desire to be healthy. And grant that I might attain that goal, to your glory and my own good. In Jesus' name, Amen.

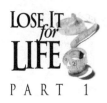

DAY 4:
Looking Below the Surface

When you keep a journal, you should look for these three eating patterns: grazing, overeating, and binge eating.

Looking at Your *Life*

Keeping a food journal provides you with an objective view of your eating patterns.

What adjectives would you use to describe your current eating habits? (For example, "unpredictable," "insatiable," and so forth)

_____

_____

_____

When during the day or week was your appetite "biggest"? When was it smaller? Why?

_____

_____

_____

Physical hunger is not what motivates grazing. You eat because food is available or because it sounds good at the time.

Picture a cow grazing all day chewing grass. We know that's not a flattering visual but that picture is similar to what some overeaters do—they graze all day on food—a little here and there. Never really eating huge amounts at once, but continuously eating though out the day. How much a part of your daily routine is grazing?

_____

_____

_____

Overeating is when you eat past a feeling of being full or to the point of feeling uncomfortable. Maybe you wolf down three servings quickly, or you keep going back to the buffet.

What's behind this habit? When do you see this tendency in yourself?

_____

_____

_____

Binge eating involves uncontrolled eating episodes in which you consume a large number of calories in a short amount of time. Usually bingeing is done in secret. It happens when you are alone, and it ends in disgust and a very uncomfortable physical feeling.

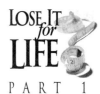

If you are a binger, describe how it makes you feel. (If you are not, speculate on why this habit has so many in its grip.)

_____

_____

Use your food journal as an objective information source for the purpose of helping you identify your overeating habits. At this point in the weight loss journey, it's best not to judge your eating by subjective feelings. You simply can't trust them to be accurate. Remember, *those who consistently record food intake, lose weight.*

Learning a New Way of *Life*

One of the greatest myths people believe is that losing weight guarantees happiness. It's true that shedding extra pounds does make people feel better on the outside. But losing weight can also uncover more than we sometimes imagine.

The authors cite the following letter from a woman named Cathy:

> This week has been a rough one. Lately I've been thinking about the past through rose-colored glasses. Somehow, I remember being happier and more jovial at 350 pounds. I remember being a social butterfly—loud, crazy, and extremely talkative—always looking for spontaneous fun! Sort of like a female "John Candy." Boy, have I changed! Without the white stuff (sugar), my personality now is nothing like the one I describe.
>
> Bottom line: I have somehow manipulated my memories into believing that being fat was fun, and I know this isn't true. I guess I'm looking for a good reason to sabotage my new healthy lifestyle. I need help on this one!

What examples can you think of in your life of a "good thing" resulting in consequences that were different than you expected?

_____

_____

Emotionally, binge eating leads to feelings of depression, anxiety, low self-esteem, powerlessness, anger, fear, numbness, social withdrawal and isolation.

When people shed weight—especially a lot of weight—other issues begin to surface. Keeping the weight off requires changes in thinking and doing. For example, speculate on the experience of the person who has always used food to numb unpleasant feelings from the past, but who now refuses to use food as a crutch.

How might such a person be tempted to sabotage his or her success?

_____

_____

35

LOSE IT
for
LIFE

PART 1

What is the best solution to overcoming such inner tension?

_____

_____

Our food-obsessed lifestyles may not be healthy, but they surely are familiar and comfortable. As we peel away the weight, we also peel away our old defenses. What's left is the reality we have feared facing. For many overweight people, the past is full of hurtful experiences that were never resolved.

The authors argue that unresolved hurts are usually the root reasons why people begin to overeat in the first place, and that they can be healed. What do you think of this argument?

_____

_____

What have been the great wounding incidents in your life? Be honest. Remember, Jesus said the truth would set us free.

_____

_____

_____

Read Isaiah 61:2–3. This great passage shows God's desire to send a Savior who will heal his defeated, disillusioned people and fill them with hope:

> *God sent me to announce the year of his grace—a celebration of God's destruction of our enemies—and to comfort all who mourn, To care for the needs of all who mourn in Zion, give them bouquets of roses instead of ashes, Messages of joy instead of news of doom, a praising heart instead of a languid spirit. Rename them "Oaks of Righteousness" planted by God to display his glory (THE MESSAGE).*

Listen. Be still before the Lord. What is God saying to you in this passage?

_____

_____

_____

Losing It for *Life*

Cathy's choices may be yours as well.

- Am I going to push ahead, despite the pain that will surface as I remember the past—without using food to cover it up?
- Will I seek other God-honoring ways to cope with my present stress?
- Will I go back to my old habit of numbing out bad feelings?

What kinds of feelings, questions, and concerns do those choices stir in you?

_____

_____

_____

Dr. Linda remembers being in church as a child and learning and singing a chorus that went: "I'm in right, out right, upright, down right, happy all the time. Since Jesus Christ came in and cleansed my heart from sin, I'm in right, out right, upright, downright happy all the time."

How accurately does that picture life as a Christian? Explain.

_____

_____

_____

If we choose to confront the reality of our lives, we won't feel happy all the time. We will have to learn to deal with difficulty and affliction. We may have to grieve losses of not having the perfect family, of a disappointing marriage, of children making bad choices, of critical and controlling bosses, and so forth. But we will learn to move past those hurts, no longer needing food as a cover up.

Hebrews 12:2 says: "Let us fix our eyes on Jesus, the author and perfecter of our faith, who for the joy set before him endured the cross, scorning its shame, and sat down at the right hand of the throne of God." In the short-term, what was Jesus called by God to experience?

_____

_____

_____

Because He was willing to endure short-term pain, what did Jesus ultimately receive?

_____

_____

_____

What does Jesus' example suggest with regard to your own experience and path? Why is embarking on the LIFL plan worth it long-term?

_____

_____

_____

LOSE It
for
LIFE
PART 1

You can learn to tolerate bad feelings, walk through them, and let go of them. Walk through the pain; don't avoid it.

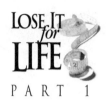

DAY 5:
Lose the Unrealistic Expectations

PART 1

Thinking your life will be totally happy if you lose weight is only one of many unrealistic expectations concerning weight loss. Reevaluating your expectations is necessary. It's part of accepting reality. Our goal in this workbook session is to uncover other wrong ways of thinking. Are you ready?

Looking at Your *Life*

Belief #1: All I have to do is lose weight. Nothing more will be required.

What is fallacious or dangerous about this kind of thinking?

_____

_____

In addition to the "what" of weight gain, why must we also focus on the "why"?

_____

_____

Belief #2: All kinds of opportunities will come to me when I lose weight.

When have you ever fallen victim to thinking that your life would be awash with good if you lost weight, only to be disappointed when it didn't turn out that way?

_____

_____

What do you think about the idea that blossoming friendships, a better marriage, a more active dating life, and so forth have less to do with losing weight and more to do with how you act and feel about yourself?

_____

_____

Belief #3: I will like myself better when I'm thinner.

To this idea, the authors cry: "Reality check! Red pill time! You may like your self less for a short time as you confront things about yourself that need changing!" Do you agree? Why or why not?

_____

_____

Remember, being thin can take away a very comfortable excuse: "People don't like me because I'm fat." In actuality, they may avoid you because you are insensitive or something else. What concerns you as you realize that LIFL, in addition to being a weight-loss program is also a call to confront the not-so-nice parts of yourself, and make changes?

_____

_____

Belief #4: Food is my best friend. I'll be giving up a good thing.

In what specific ways is food a poor substitute for community and connection?

_____

_____

Describe a time in your life when a great meal deeply satisfied your innermost longings to be cared for emotionally and spiritually. Did it work? Did it last?

_____

_____

Belief #5: I must be perfect for God to work in me.

How does holding onto this belief cause us to cover up problems and be dishonest about our struggles?

_____

_____

Learning a New Way of *Life*

Our souls have a great enemy called Satan or the devil. He is described in the Bible as a liar and a murderer (John 8:44), as the ruler of this age who blinds people to truth (2 Corinthians 4:4), as an accuser of God's people (Revelation 12:10), and as one who is like a roaring lion, intent on destroying lives (1 Peter 5:8). Ephesians 6 speaks of the reality of spiritual warfare against this brutal adversary and of the importance of taking up the armor of God to fend off the evil one's diabolical attacks.

How would you say Satan most effectively wars against you—using food and eating?

_____

_____

Where are the chinks in your armor? Where are his fiery arrows landing in your life?

_____

_____

_____

When we wallow in guilt and shame from our past, we basically tell God that His Son's sacrifice didn't matter. He's taken all your guilt and shame to the cross, where Jesus died for our sin, and He doesn't

It's never too late with God. God doesn't hold grudges. He forgives you and invites you to be His, with every cellulite wrinkle and flaw.

LOSE IT
for
LIFE
PART 1

*The truth
transforms us,
but we have to
cooperate in
the process in
order to look
like the Christ,
who does the
transforming.*

want you holding on to it. He says, "I'll take your failures and build your future." And He has a great one planned for you. Do you dare believe this? Respond honestly.

_____

_____

Before His death, Jesus knew that Peter would deny him three times. He knew Peter would fail miserably. Read John 21. What do you see there? How does Jesus use Peter's failures and redeem his losses? How do you think Peter felt before, during, and after this encounter?

_____

_____

Read John 8:31–32. Before the truth can set us free, what must we be willing to do? (See also James 1:22.)

_____

_____

The authors argue that we see so little genuine transformation in our churches because the church often penalizes us for being honest. We hide our problems, as we are encouraged to put on a happy face.

Do you agree with that assessment? What do you think would happen if the people in your church knew all your stuff—your past, your hurts, your wrong choices, your failures?

_____

_____

In the Bible, we find unflattering details of all kinds of biblical characters. What does this suggest about God, His power, His grace, and our future?

_____

_____

Losing It for *Life*

Unfortunately, often we *are* judged by our weight. If we are heavy, many people will conclude we lack will power and self-discipline. Haven't you heard, "Well, just stop putting the food in your mouth!"? And don't you always want to scream back, "If it were that easy, I'd be at my ideal weight right now!" The lesson? We won't always find the acceptance we desire from others. We can't control what people think or say.

Given this harsh reality, how can we go on? Where do we find acceptance and support?

_____

_____

In light of all the insensitive, impatient people, how can we trust that a few people *will* prove to be faithful friends and comrades on the LIFL journey?

_____

_____

How do we guard against the ever-present temptation of letting the opinions of others be our motivation for losing weight?

_____

_____

The authors recommend a prayer along these lines:

> *God, I refuse to accept those words of being lazy, ugly, out-of-control, (fill in the blank) as definitions of who I am. With Your help, I will discover the true me. You created me and declared Your creation good. Amen.*

Why is it important to know who we are in Christ? How does someone develop a biblical self-image?

_____

_____

_____

You are not what you weigh. You have worth just because God created you.

Based on what you've read here so far, how does this weight-loss/weight-management plan differ from others that you have tried?

_____

_____

What would you like to see God do in your life—not just in your body but also in your heart in the months and years to come?

_____

_____

_____

Remembering that there are no quick fixes or instant solutions, what is your plan for when you encounter hard times on this journey?

_____

_____

Preparation: Read chapter three of Lose It for Life *before you begin the lessons for Week 3.*

DAY 1:
Why Dieting Doesn't Work

LOSE IT
for
LIFE

PART 1

*Seven Keys
to Lose it
for Life*

We can't think of anything more depressing than dieting. Who wants to willingly embark on a life of deprivation and eating foods you don't enjoy? Just mentioning the word "diet" is depressing. We can almost hear your groans and moans, "Not another diet!"

Looking at Your *Life*

What was your very first diet? What eventually happened?

_____

_____

_____

*We don't want
you to diet.
Lose the word
from your
vocabulary.*

Describe your most recent dieting experience.

_____

_____

_____

In what situations are you most prone to graze? (Check all that apply.)

_____ when I am lonely
_____ when I am bored
_____ when I am anxious/stressed
_____ when I am afraid
_____ when I am idle
_____ whenever food is readily available
_____ from the time I wake up until the time I hit the hay
_____ when I am _____

Learning a New Way of *Life*

You'd think we would have it figured out by now. But we don't. Dieting is inherently frustrating because it actually gets us to obsess over food. We end up craving whatever foods the diet forbids us to have. It's not so much "forbidden fruit" as forbidden *sweets* or *starches* or *fatty fare.* We become transfixed by and preoccupied with whatever is off limits. It's only a matter of time until the siren call of some sinful delicacy wears down our willpower. Can we get a witness?

Because of our past dietary failures and personal hurts, these are the kinds of beliefs we find rattling around in our heads and hearts:

"You're disgusting. Can't you even get it right for one day?"
"Why even try? You know you're going to fail. It's just a matter of time."

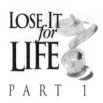

LOSE IT for LIFE

PART 1

"You? Thin? Who are you kidding?"

"How many times have you tried to lose weight? A thousand? Two thousand?"

"Why don't you just face facts? You're fat and you'll always be fat."

Write down some messages of the "tapes" that play in your mind.

_____

_____

_____

Consider the following passages of Scripture. These are not nice ideas or warm wishes. They are declarations of eternal, divine truth. God doesn't force us to believe these statements, but if we do—if we base our identity and worth on these biblical precepts—we begin to view God, the world, and ourselves differently. And over time, we begin to act differently (see Romans 12:1–2).

The thief comes only to steal and kill and destroy; I have come that they may have life, and have it to the full (John 10:10).

How great is the love the Father has lavished on us, that we should be called children of God! And that is what we are! (1 John 3:1).

For we are God's masterpiece. He has created us anew in Christ Jesus, so that we can do the good things he planned for us long ago (Ephesians 2:10, THE MESSAGE).

Now to him who is able to do immeasurably more than all we ask or imagine, according to his power that is at work within us (Ephesians 3:20).

For God did not give us a spirit of timidity, but a spirit of power, of love and of self-discipline (2 Timothy 1:7).

According to these verses, what is the truth about you?

_____

_____

_____

LIFL Reminders:
- You don't need a new diet; you need a new mindset and lifestyle.
- Remove unhealthy food temptations from your household.
- Drink a lot of water. It's good for you and it can take the edge off your cravings!
- Eat smaller portions and eat slowly.

- Get your body moving.
- Find stress relievers and "emptiness fillers" other than food: cleaning, exercise, serving others, calling friends, yard work, taking a hot shower, and others.

Losing It for *Life*

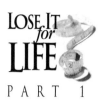

Let's look more closely at why dieting usually ends in disaster and disillusionment.

Check the boxes by the following statements with which you have firsthand experience.

❑ Dieting means deprivation.

The cycle of depriving yourself, then giving in, then feeling guilty which leads to more overeating, is classic. It doesn't work and leads to feelings of failure and shame. And it certainly doesn't address the reasons *why* you overeat in the first place.

The authors observe: "Diets make food your enemy. And as the dietitians remind us, 'There are no forbidden foods.' Anything in moderation will not make you fat! . . . When we deprive ourselves from certain foods, chances are we'll binge or overeat." Do you agree or disagree with these statements? Why?

_____

_____

_____

❑ Dieting doesn't fill the empty place.

Many people overeat because they have emotional needs or want something. But as much as they try, food doesn't fill those empty spaces.

Think of a recent experience (for example, a rejection, a slight, a disappointment, and so forth) in which you reacted by turning to food for comfort. What happened? How were you feeling as you ate? What about afterwards?

_____

_____

_____

Be honest. Do you look to God when you are swamped by feelings of emptiness? Why or why not?

_____

_____

_____

Sometimes overeating is triggered because we feel "empty." We have no active, alive life with God. We don't trust Him to help us handle our difficult feelings and so we eat to fill the void.

LOSE IT for LIFE
PART 1

Thinking you are going to miss something sets you up to overeat. What you can't have, you want. This idea goes all the way back to the Garden of Eden.

You always have a choice to eat a food, eat less of it or skip it entirely. A little of something may satisfy your want.

❏ **Dieting means missing something.**

We often hunt down foods and eat like a condemned criminal having his or her last meal. How prone are you to fall into this kind of thinking? What foods do you find practically irresistible?

_____

_____

_____

❏ **Dieting gives the control to others instead of you.**

The diet is like big brother watching your every move. Add the myriad expert voices telling you to eat only low-fat, high protein, low carbs, high carbs, only vegetables. . . . It's enough to make a person throw in the towel.

If maturity means being responsible for your own choices, then what does it say when we rush out and buy every new dieting book that hits the bookshelves?

_____

_____

_____

❏ **Dieting sets up bingeing.**

To illustrate this point, the authors tell the story of a salesman named Jim (see the story in chapter three of the book).

With what in Jim's experience do you relate?

_____

_____

What is the most helpful truth you've discovered in this lesson? Why?

_____

_____

_____

DAY 2:
A Proper View of Eating

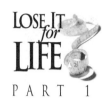

LOSE IT
for
LIFE

P A R T   1

Since we find so much distortion in our culture concerning food, it's best to look at God's original intention for eating. First, think about your own view of food.

Looking at Your *Life*

When you were a child, how was food treated or used in your household? For instance, were desserts and treats used a reward? Was the withholding of food used as a punishment? Was food offered as a way of "cheering up" after a bad experience?

_____

_____

What are your most vivid childhood memories of food?

_____

_____

God created us with a physical need to eat and provided food as a way to satisfy that need.

Estimate how much time you spend (on average) weekly in each of the following areas:

_____ planning meals/thinking about what to cook or eat
_____ buying food/grocery shopping
_____ stocking /rearranging food in the pantry/refrigerator
_____ cooking/preparing food
_____ actually eating meals (at home or dining out)
_____ waiting to get your food (either in a restaurant or a fast food drive-through lane)
_____ cleaning up after meals
_____ talking about food (good recipes, what you're going to eat, what you did eat, etc.)
_____ snacking

What's your total? Does that seem about right? Excessive? What conclusions can you draw from this exercise?

_____

_____

We don't often hear teaching or sermons on food or eating in a way that honors God. Why is this subject, which is such a major part of every day life, so seldom talked about or thought about from a biblical perspective?

_____

_____

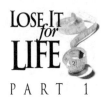

PART 1

Learning a New Way of *Life*

Let's take a quick and broad overview of food as mentioned in the Bible. Eating and drinking were major ingredients of fellowship and hospitality in biblical days. People held feasts, celebrated weddings, invited others for meals, cooked for guests, and used food to nourish, strengthen, and celebrate.

What are your favorite social occasions or holidays that involve big meals? Why?

_____

_____

Food figures prominently in the Bible. The first temptation and sin involved eating; the ending involves a great marriage banquet.

In the Old Testament, God prescribed seven feasts for the Israelites. These were both solemn assemblies and times of great celebration, intended to commemorate God's deliverance of Israel from Egypt and His constant care in the wilderness. Eating also figured prominently in the sacrificial system that God instructed His people to follow. The Promised Land was assessed largely on the basis of its fruitfulness (that is, its ability to provide rich supplies of food).

When the Israelites wandered in the wilderness, God provided manna from heaven—a supernatural supply of daily food (see Exodus 16). What was God trying to teach His people?

_____

_____

The New Testament recorded that Jesus ate meals with his disciples (including the Last Supper), shared a meal with Lazarus, and had dinner cooked by Martha. Preaching in Lystra, the apostle Paul exclaimed: "[God] has shown kindness by giving you rain from heaven and crops in their seasons; he provides you with plenty of food and fills your hearts with joy" (Acts 14:17).

When teaching His followers how to pray, why do you think Jesus included the petition found in Matthew 6:11?

_____

_____

What conclusions can we therefore draw about food and eating?

_____

_____

Food and drink were often a major focal point of miracles—Jesus turned water into wine at a wedding and fed thousands with loaves and fishes on hillsides. In Mark, Jesus compared the coming of His kingdom to a wedding feast. Throughout the Bible, food is discussed symbolically as well as literally and is enjoyed and celebrated.

The resurrected Christ grilled fish on the beach and enjoyed this simple meal with His disciples. He didn't *have* to do this and yet He did. Why, do you think?

_____

_____

In the book of Revelation, the apostle John was given a glimpse into the future at the end of this world. John said, "And I saw an angel standing in the sun, who cried in a loud voice to all the birds flying in midair, 'Come, gather together for the great supper of God'" (Revelation 19:17). What do you imagine this supper will be like?

_____

_____

Losing It for *Life*

It is important to have a healthy perspective about food. As physical beings, we need nourishment—vitamins and minerals, "fuel" to run our human bodies. There is nothing intrinsically wrong or sinful with food. Yet, like all of God's good gifts—rest, wealth, sex, and so forth—food can be abused, misused, or turned into a god. Our goal here is to develop a healthy, biblical perspective on food and eating.

If you had to summarize what God's Word says about food in a few broad principles, how would you do so? Write your summary principles here.

1.

2.

3.

4.

5.

First Corinthians 10:31 says, "So whether you eat or drink or whatever you do, do it all for the glory of God." How does someone eat for the "glory of God"?

_____

_____

Think about your eating habits for the last couple of days, weeks, or years. In what ways have you glorified God in your attitudes and actions surrounding food? In what specific ways have you not?

_____

_____

"The LORD Almighty will prepare a feast of rich food for all peoples, a banquet of aged wine— the best of meats and the finest of wines" (Isaiah 25:6).

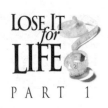

PART 1

DAY 3:
What Is Gluttony?

As with most human activities, we can eat and drink to excess. The biblical term for having a ravenous and unrestrained appetite is *gluttony*. A glutton is defined as someone who gorges on food and who is marked by excessive desire. Let's look at what can we learn from Scripture about gluttony, a topic rarely discussed in the American modern church.

The reason we need to understand gluttony is that it can impede our spiritual progress, keeping us from enjoying a victorious spiritual life.

Looking at Your *Life*

When have you heard the word "glutton" used in regular conversation?

_____

_____

When does normal, healthy eating cross over into the realm of gluttony?

_____

_____

Check any of the following that you personally regard as gluttony:

_____ eating three big meals a day

_____ making more than one trip to the food bar

_____ eating to the point of feel stuffed

_____ eating more than a certain amount of calories in a day

_____ having frantic late-night binges

_____ super-sizing meals at fast-food restaurants

_____ cleaning one's plate—and also perhaps eating the "leftovers" off a spouse's or child's plate

_____ having two scoops instead of one

_____ going back for seconds

_____ inhaling the meal in a very short time

_____ eating out of a container or out of the serving dish

_____ other:

What are your specific criteria for knowing when you've crossed the line into gluttony? (Note: If you don't have any, now might be a good time to take a shot at creating a set of guidelines for knowing when too much of a good thing is too much.)

_____

_____

_____

Learning a New Way of *Life*

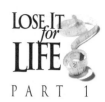

One of the Bible's direct references to gluttony is found in Proverbs 23, a chapter about the importance of exercising restraint. In Proverbs 23:2–3, Solomon instructs, "Don't gobble your food; don't talk with your mouth full. And don't stuff yourself; bridle your appetite" (THE MESSAGE). In verse 21 of that same chapter, he states, "Drunks and gluttons will end up on skid row, in a stupor and dressed in rags."

How would you summarize the message of these verses?

_____

_____

Jesus talked about how the people tried to discredit His claims to be the promised Messiah by calling Him a glutton. "And I, the Son of Man, feast and drink, and you say, 'He's a glutton and a drunkard, and a friend of the worst sort of sinners!' but wisdom is shown to be right by what results from it" (Matthew 11:19 NLT).

What does this passage reveal about:

     Jesus Christ?

_____

     eating and drinking?

_____

In the above instance, gluttony was viewed as a negative behavior trait. Feasting was not a problem, but becoming a lush was. And a lush is not a positive description of anyone. The intent was to criticize Jesus by calling Him a glutton and drunkard—someone who couldn't bridle His appetite or exercise control over His life. Isn't it crazy that the Pharisees applied these labels to Christ? He's God. He's always been in total control of His passions and desires.

Imagine a life free from gluttonous behavior. What would it be like to live moderately? To be free to taste and enjoy a small bit of anything, without going overboard? How—long-term—would such a practice change your daily existence?

_____

_____

Losing It for *Life*

Deuteronomy 21:18–21 weaves together the concepts of gluttony and rebellion. Ponder these verses:

> *"When a man has a stubborn son, a real rebel who won't do a thing his mother and*
> *father tell him, and even though they discipline him he still won't obey, his father and*

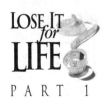

P A R T   1

Gluttony is one of the so-called "Seven Deadly Sins"—because it can be harmful to one's relationship with God and others.

mother shall forcibly bring him before the leaders at the city gate and say to the city fathers, 'This son of ours is a stubborn rebel; he won't listen to a thing we say. He's a glutton and a drunk'"(The Message).

Amazingly, the punishment for this type of rebellion was stoning—to death! (The Bible records no instances of parents having done this.) The consequence was meant to deter rebellion. The point here isn't to suggest an extreme model for dealing with rebellious children. *Please* don't apply it that way! We believe, however, that Deuteronomy 21 highlights a broad, important principle—rebellion (against authority, whether parental, civil, or eternal) ultimately leads to destruction and negative consequences, consequences that God wanted the children of Israel to avoid for their own good.

Do you eat when you want to rebel? Or when you want to get back at someone—at a spouse, a parent, at God? Are you living a compliant life on the outside but secretly rebelling against something or someone on the inside?

_____

_____

_____

Whether we eat in a passive-aggressive fashion, to lash out or punish someone else, or we eat frantically, out of some irrational fear that we might miss out on "our fair share," gluttony is sin.

Read 1 John 1:9. In your own words, what does it say?

_____

_____

_____

In some cases, angry rebellion is a motive for overeating.

To *confess* means literally to "say the same thing." When we confess our sin, we agree with what God says about it. So, what *does* God say about our sins? First, He says they are an affront to His holy character and standard (Romans 3:23). Second, He says that in Christ our sins are forgiven—all of them (Colossians 2:13). Third, because of the new nature Christ gives us (2 Corinthians 5:17) when we trust Him, sin has no more power over us. We do not have to keep giving in to the same temptations (see Romans 6)!

In light of these truths, write out a full confession to God of any acts of gluttony. Claim His promise of complete forgiveness and cleansing.

_____

_____

_____

DAY 4:
Our Bodies for the Glory of God

As you read through the biblical references to gluttony, you can understand why more ministers don't preach on this topic! It seems negative and depressing, but it isn't. God created your body. He chose you as His own child. His Spirit lives inside you. Let's explore in this session what it means that our bodies are to be used for the glory of God.

Looking at Your *Life*

Some troubled youths cut themselves, a practice referred to as "self-mutilation." What do you think motivates this strange practice against one's body?

_____

_____

The number of people who are choosing to undergo cosmetic surgery is skyrocketing. Why is this one of the biggest growth industries in the western world?

_____

_____

This may be difficult or painful exercise. Take some time think about how you view your body. What do you like about it? Dislike? What body parts or physical features would you change instantly if you could? Why?

_____

_____

"Don't you know that your body is the temple of the Holy Spirit, who lives in you and was given to you by God? You do not belong to yourself, for God bought you with a high price. So you must honor God with your body" (1 Corinthians 6:19–20).

Learning a New Way of *Life*

The shocking claim of the gospel is that God Himself took on human form. The Creator came into His creation in the person of Christ. For thirty-plus years Jesus lived with all the constraints of a human body. How does this fact encourage you?

_____

_____

In a messianic passage referring to the coming Christ, Isaiah 53:2 says, "There was nothing beautiful or majestic about his appearance, nothing to attract us to him." How do you respond to this description of Christ?

_____

_____

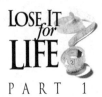

LOSE IT for LIFE

PART 1

In Psalm 139, David seems to exult in his body (that is, the precise way God had made him). "You . . . knit me together in my mother's womb. Thank you for making me so wonderfully complex! Your workmanship is marvelous—and how well I know it" (NLT). Is this how you view yourself? Why or why not?

_____

_____

When we give our ultimate attention and affection to something— even food—we are guilty of idolatry.

Our bodies are the dwelling place of the Most High God (1 Corinthians 6:19–20). What does this suggest about how we treat and take care of our bodies? What kinds of things are appropriate? What kinds of things are inappropriate?

_____

_____

Matthew 6:25 says: "If you decide for God, living a life of God-worship, it follows that you don't fuss about what's on the table at mealtimes or whether the clothes in your closet are in fashion. There is far more to your life than the food you put in your stomach, more to your outer appearance than the clothes you hang on your body" (THE MESSAGE).

In what ways can our modern preoccupation with food become a kind of "idolatry"?

_____

_____

Losing It for *Life*

When we become preoccupied with what we will eat, when we look forward to meals more than concentrating on knowing and loving and serving God, we are out of balance. Whenever we get absorbed or obsessed with what we are going to eat, how much we'll be able to have, and how often we can get it, we have ceased following Christ.

Read Matthew 6:33. What does this passage say about:
Your priorities?

_____

God's care for those who have right priorities?

_____

A person who decides to be a Christ-follower has the promise that God will meet physical needs as well as emotional and spiritual ones. How can you realistically and practically accept those promises right now—and begin to enjoy them?

_____

Let's say after these last few workbook sessions, you have realized a tendency towards gluttony. Perhaps you habitually overeat. Or you fantasize excessively about food. Or you have let your body, the temple of the living God, get to an unhealthy state. What does all this mean? Does God look upon you with disgust? (Hint: See Romans 8:31–39.)

_____

_____

Please understand. You are not condemned by God or by the LIFL community for overeating. God only desires to bring you to improved health, to remove your obsession with food, to prevent negative consequences related to overeating, and to help you enjoy meals and fellowship with others. He wants you to experience the enjoyment of food, the pleasure of taste, and the sensation of a full stomach rather than be bound by guilt, physically discomfort, or negative health consequences related to obesity and bingeing.

The Bible offers the following solutions for idolatry and excess. Spend a few final moments thinking about each of these statements and jotting down any questions, thoughts, or insights you have.

- We get out of spiritual poverty by developing *self-control*, a fruit of the Spirit (see Galatians 5:22).

How developed is this trait in you?

_____

_____

_____

- We are called to practice balance and moderation in all things, "Moderation is better than muscle, self-control better than political power" (Proverbs 16:32, THE MESSAGE).

In what areas of your life do you see victory and balance?

_____

_____

_____

- A transformed life begins with absolute surrender (see Romans 12:1).

What are some signs that a person has truly surrendered his or her life to God?

_____

_____

_____

LOSE IT
for
LIFE

PART 1

God wants balance in your life—so go ahead, enjoy eating. Just do not become a glutton. Anything taken to excess can block a vibrant relationship with God. Moderation is key.

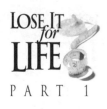

PART 1

DAY 5:
Distinguishing the Hungers

What is hunger? As part of our ongoing effort to lose it for life, we must know the difference between physical, emotional, and spiritual hunger. The three are very different and often confused. Let's explore in more detail.

We have other needs and desires, apart from those of our physical bodies. Among those are the needs to be safe, to belong, to be loved, to be esteemed, and to grow.

Looking at Your *Life*

Speaking of hunger, one person admitted:

> I eat but I'm not really hungry. At least I don't think I am. I'm not really sure. Sometimes I feel like I could eat everything in the cupboards, like I'm ravenous. So I just do. I never really think about if I'm hungry or not. I think, *I just really like food, lots of food.* And lots of times, I crave things—like cookies. I'll go to the bakery and pretend to be buying a dozen cookies for my kids at school, but really, I plan on eating them all.

In what ways can you relate to this kind of hunger, this kind of craving?

_____

_____

When do you experience it most?

_____

_____

Write briefly about a time in your life when you felt spiritually ravenous—when you were hungry to know God?

_____

_____

Write briefly about a recent time when you felt starved for emotional connection, when loneliness hit you intensely. What did you do?

_____

_____

Learning a New Way of *Life*

Physical hunger is normal, a natural God-given sensation and a cue that our human bodies needs refueling.

What is the hungriest you can ever remember being? Put another way, what is the longest period you've ever gone without food? Describe that time.

_____

_____

What are the indicators of true physical hunger?

_____

_____

How would you define "emotional hunger"? What are the symptoms of this common phenomenon?

_____

_____

In the LIFL book, the authors distinguish between physical hunger and emotional hunger.

Physical Hunger	**Emotional Hunger**
Builds gradually	Hits suddenly, "starving"
Stomach starts to rumble and growl	Anxiety; but no real "physical" symptom of feeling hungry
Feel full and you stop eating	Overeat even if feel full
Different foods will satisfy	Crave very specific foods; nothing else satisfies
Physically feel empty in pit of stomach	Mouth and mind are tasting the food
Need to eat but can wait	Eat now to ease whatever is happening
Eat and feel fine	Eat (often excessively) and feel guilt and shame
4–5 hours since last meal; feel light-headed, low energy	Upset and want to eat now
Choose foods purposefully	Automatic or absentminded eating

Where do you see yourself (your own experience and habits) in this chart?

_____

_____

When do you tend to be an emotional eater? In what ways?

_____

_____

Food is used like a drug—distracting, numbing, and helping us avoid the reality of hurt and pain or the emptiness of an unmet need.

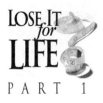

During the Sermon on the Mount, Jesus said, "Blessed are you who hunger now, for you will be satisfied" (Luke 17:21). The Greek word for *hunger* is *peinas*, meaning "to be hungry," to be famished, to be starved. What does it mean to hunger for God? What does it look like and feel like to be satisfied in God?

_____

_____

The authors suggest that often we are spiritually starving but don't feed our hunger the right way. We become distracted with and chase after other things that can't and won't fill that spiritual void. In what ways and at what stages in your life has this been your experience?

_____

_____

_____

Author Beth Moore says, "Victory is not determined as much by what we've been delivered *from* as by what we've been delivered *to*." You won't be victorious over food and overeating eating unless you look to God to satisfy you. Nothing else will really do. God wants to deliver you from the need to overeat. He wants you to find your purpose, move in His power, and live a life of overcoming. His way of doing that is to offer Himself to you. He is your deliverer. He offers relationship, intimacy, and abundant life, peace, joy and so much more. The "more" He offers will satisfy. Listen, He wants you, chose you, and is waiting to fill your mouth with good things.

What do these words and claims stir in you?

_____

_____

_____

The following Scriptures speak of the great hope we have in Christ:

> *For everything that was written in the past was written to teach us, so that through endurance and the encouragement of the Scriptures we might have hope (Romans 15:4).*

> *May the God of hope fill you with all joy and peace as you trust in him, so that you may overflow with hope by the power of the Holy Spirit (Romans 15:13).*

> *I pray also that the eyes of your heart may be enlightened in order that you may know the hope to which he has called you, the riches of his glorious inheritance in the saints (Ephesians 1:18).*

What would it be like to overflow with hope? How do you think you'd be different if you developed and maintained a rich, intimate daily walk with Jesus?

_____

_____

Losing It for *Life*

Every time we eat, certain "triggers" or "signals" precede our eating. For example, a physical trigger is usually something like a rumbling stomach, a headache, dizziness, weakness, or low energy. Some common emotional triggers are feeling upset, bored, hurt, angry, disappointed, lonely, happy, and so forth.

By learning to distinguish these various cues, we begin to get a handle on our eating. One way to do this is to keep a record. Remember, a big component of the LIFL plan is using a food journal to document what we eat, when we eat it, and why we do so.

As you develop this habit, you are asked to try to describe the motive for your eating. If you notice that many of your daily eating episodes stem from emotional hunger, then we have work to do. The goal of LIFL is to learn to eat in response to physical cues, not emotional ones.

The next time you eat, take a guess at which type of hunger you are experiencing. List the three columns shown below.

• In the first column, check which hunger you think you are having.

• In the second column, record your feelings, physical sensations, emotions, and thoughts right before you wanted to eat.

• In the third column, write how you felt after you ate. Read what you listed and decide if you checked the correct hunger.

A blank copy of this chart is provided in Appendix B of the *Lose It for Life* book. Here's an example.

What we often think is hunger for food or even emotional hunger may actually be a hunger for more of God!

Physical hunger	Emotional hunger	Before I ate, I felt: *(list feelings and thoughts)*	After I ate, I felt: *(list feelings, physical sensations, and thoughts)*
❑	☒	upset and frustrated, wanted to eat immediately	uncomfortable
☒	❑	light-headed (last food was four hours before); stomach growling	satisfied and energized

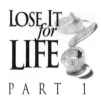

PART 1

The important thing is to discover exactly what triggers you to overeat. Write these cues down and study them.

If you aren't sure what you are feeling or thinking when you eat, focus on the experience of eating and try to become attuned to your physical and emotional state. The goal is to stay in the moment of eating and avoid the common habit of eating without thinking. Here's an additional exercise to try:

- Sixty seconds before you eat, sit quietly (no distractions) and think: *What am I feeling and what am I thinking about right now?* Record this.
- Then look at what you are about to eat. Notice how it tastes. *Do you like what you are eating? Do you like the feel of it in your mouth? How does it feel in your stomach?*
- After you finish, take another sixty seconds and write down how you feel—energized, tired, unsatisfied, content, etc.

This short exercise will put you in touch with the experience of eating. It will slow you down and help you pay attention to all the sensations involved in eating. Many times after emotional eating, you'll feel tired and sluggish or won't feel satisfied. That's because eating wasn't what you needed to do. In addition, when you choose sugary foods, your blood sugar rises and falls, which makes you feel tired. The goal is to stop eating when you aren't physically hungry, and stop stuffing food in when you are upset or feeling emotional.

The authors offer this encouragement:

> God has so much more for you. He doesn't want you dragging through life being defeated by your weight. He wants to give you good things—more of His power, more of His Spirit, more of His love and compassion. The urgency you feel to fill up with food, to overeat, could be the Holy Spirit urging you to satisfy your spiritual hunger through God. Are you afraid you won't get what you need? Not to worry. God has enough to go around for all of us. His resources are limitless. He is the Living Water that never runs dry. He is the Bread of Life who promises eternal life. The fullness He has for you cannot be found in the temporal things of this world. And once you experience His fullness, you'll never hunger again!

Hunger for more of God. God is the originator and giver of all true satisfaction. Perhaps you've tried to find satisfaction in many other ways. Nothing completely fulfills but more of God. Spiritual hunger is a good because, like little birds, God is waiting for us to open our mouths so that He can fill them.

Do you dare believe these promises? Write out a prayer below that expresses your spiritual hunger. Offer it sincerely to God. Then take a few simple steps of faith.

_____

_____

_____

Preparation: Read chapter four of Lose It for Life *before you begin the lessons for Week 4.*

DAY 1:
The Unique You

Our goal isn't merely losing weight; it is keeping it off and embracing a healthier overall lifestyle. To do that, we need to think through the various *physical* influences and factors that affect weight loss and general health. That's our goal for these five workbook lessons.

Looking at Your *Life*

Early on we mentioned that "one size does not fit all." Your physical body is unique and your one-of-a-kind individuality must be factored in. Any successful eating/exercise plan will have to be tailored specifically for you.

Take a few minutes to do a little family medical history and weight assessment. What are some of the health issues or diseases that have cropped up in your immediate and extended family?

_____

_____

What close relatives struggle with their weight?

_____

_____

In your opinion, who is the healthiest individual in your immediate or extended family? What are his or her eating habits and exercise rituals?

_____

_____

Which parent are you most like in your body shape/type?

_____

_____

Let's broaden that parental comparison. Put a check mark by which parent you most resemble in the following categories:

Dad	Mom	Both	Neither	Category
____	____	____	____	basic temperament/personality
____	____	____	____	personal preferences
____	____	____	____	social skills
____	____	____	____	hobbies/leisure pursuits

LOSE IT
for
LIFE

PART 1

*Seven Keys
to Lose it
for Life*

If you have a family history of obesity, you have a greater chance of being obese. This doesn't doom you to be over-weight, but it is an influence you should recognize.

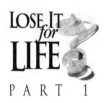

LOSE IT *for* **LIFE**

PART 1

Your genetic history is part of who you are. But it's not so much the hand you are dealt, but how you play that hand that counts!

Dad	Mom	Both	Neither	Category
_____	_____	_____	_____	political views
_____	_____	_____	_____	religious/spiritual beliefs
_____	_____	_____	_____	work ethic
_____	_____	_____	_____	facial features
_____	_____	_____	_____	manner of speaking
_____	_____	_____	_____	sense of humor
_____	_____	_____	_____	good habits
_____	_____	_____	_____	bad habits
_____	_____	_____	_____	way of responding to stress
_____	_____	_____	_____	handling money
_____	_____	_____	_____	eating habits

Learning a New Way of *Life*

God's creation reveals astonishing diversity. Each person has one-of-a-kind fingerprints, distinct DNA, exclusive personal history, inimitable background, singular life experiences, and so forth.

What conclusions can we draw from this diversity? What does it say about us as human beings? About God?

_____

_____

What does this fact suggest about the way we must each approach eating, exercise, and so forth?

_____

_____

Which of your friends or acquaintances have successfully overcome an obvious family predisposition to being heavy? Call them up. Interview them. Ask them why they think they managed to avoid the family curse. Write their responses here:

_____

_____

Whatever your history or genetic picture, be aware that physical influences can speed up or slow down the work. The better informed you are, the more patient you will be with yourself when it comes to achieving your goals. Although you may not be able to control all the factors that led to being overweight, you do have control over how you respond to them.

Losing It for *Life*

Heredity plays a role in what you weigh. If you have a family history of obesity, pay special attention to your food intake and other factors that affect weight gain. Your chances of becoming obese increase by about 30 percent.[1] Researchers are still trying to decide how much of family obesity is due to shared genes or shared family eating and exercise habits. Studies of twins, however, indicate that genetic factors do account for something.

What do you know about your metabolism? What questions do you have?

_____

_____

Among other things, we inherit something called a "basal metabolic rate" (BMR). This figure is the calculated number of calories you would burn if you stayed in bed all day (a practice *not* recommended!). The lower one's BMR, the more difficult it is to lose weight. BMR is affected by height and weight (shorter folks with more fatty body tissue burn less calories). In contrast, the more lean one's body tissue, the higher the BMR. (Note: This is why the LIFL plan encourages regular, vigorous exercise—both aerobic and strength-training.) Building lean body tissue can help raise your metabolism.[2]

What are your current exercise and fitness habits?

_____

_____

In the following chart, put a check mark by the factors that raise your BMR (metabolism) and the factors that lower your BMR. (When you finish, see the answers below.)

Factor	Raises Metabolism	Lowers Metabolism
Aging	❑	❑
Fever	❑	❑
Stress	❑	❑
Heat	❑	❑
Cold	❑	❑
Fasting	❑	❑
Starving/malnutrition	❑	❑
Dieting/skipping meals	❑	❑

(Answers: Aging, fasting, starving and malnutrition lower BMR. Fever, stress, heat and cold all raise BMR.)

Why would dieting and skipping meals *lower* one's metabolism?

_____

_____

Statement: "It is better to eat one big meal every evening than to eat throughout the day." Agree or disagree? Why?

_____

_____

LOSE IT
for
LIFE

PART 1

For most people, the real culprit isn't a thyroid problem, but an overeating and under-exercising problem.

PART 1

Your biology may create more challenges. However, it won't stop you from being successful. By taking care of your body you can and will lose it for life.

BMR is also regulated by the thyroid hormone *thyroxin*. The less thyroxin produced, the lower one's metabolism. This condition *is* a problem for a small number people and may need to be checked.[3] If you suspect you have an underactive thyroid, you can have it measured by indirect calorimetry. This service is inexpensive and can easily be done at a pulmonary department at most hospitals or by sports medicine clinics.

What do you know about the role of fat cells in weight loss/management?

_____

_____

Take the following "Fat Cell True/False Quiz."

T or F?	Statement
_____	1. The number of fat cells we have and their size is a determining factor in how much we weigh and what we look like.
_____	2. In post-adolescent healthy women fat cell accumulation more or less stops—that is, there is no further increase in the number of fat cells.
_____	3. When fat cells reach their maximum size, they can divide and create more.
_____	4. Obesity results when fat cells increase in number, size or both.
_____	5. Cellulite is a common circulatory condition that changes the appearance of the deepest layers of epidermis and is treatable with skin creams.
_____	6. The number and size of fat cells reflects the amount of fat stored in the body.
_____	7. In losing weight and dieting, we actually lose some of our largest, heaviest fat cells.

*[Answers: **1.** T; **2.** T; **3.** T; **4.** T; **5.** F (When fat cells swell and become large enough to be seen through the skin—this is cellulite. As our skin gets thinner with age and less flexible, cellulite becomes more visible. The only help for this is weight loss and regular activity.[4]) **6.** T; **7.** F. (Fat cells shrink. They don't leave the body. Even if you temporarily manage to empty them, they can easily fill up and you gain weight again. This is why it is easier for someone with an excess of fat cells to gain weight.)]*

If you have a higher number of fat cells in your body, you won't lose fat cells by dieting. There is only one way to get rid of fat cells—via liposuction. This is *not* something LIFL recommends because cosmetic surgery doesn't address lifestyle changes needed.

What's the most surprising thing you've learned here? The most interesting thing?

_____

_____

DAY 2:
The Stress Factor

LOSE IT
for
LIFE

P A R T   1

You'd have to be living on another planet *not* to know that stress affects our bodies in negative ways. Sometimes when we mishandle stress, we end up misusing food—and we gain weight. Let's explore this in more detail.

While an immediate response to stress may be a loss of appetite, repeated and chronic stress can cause just the opposite.

Looking at Your *Life*

What is your best definition or description of stress?

_____

_____

What is a dictionary definition of "stress"?

_____

_____

What are the most stressful situations in your life currently? (Note: If your life is rather calm and stress-free right now, think back over the last year). You may wish to answer in terms of the following categories:

Situation	Potential Area of Stress	Specific Stressful
My finances:	❑	❑
My marriage/marital status:	❑	❑
My job/career situation:	❑	❑
My health (or lack of health):	❑	❑
My children:	❑	❑
My parents:	❑	❑
My social situation:	❑	❑
My church involvement:	❑	❑
Academic demands:	❑	❑
Other:	❑	❑

Which of the following responses are your most common reactions to stress? (Circle any or all that apply.)

I talk to friends.	I graze.	I binge.	I get angry.	I drink.
I (try to) escape.	I pray.	I complain.	I exercise.	I sleep.
I lose the urge to eat.	I shop.	I pace.	I bite my nails.	I cry.
I eat my favorite food.	I panic.	I get manic.	I throw things.	I snap.
I become controlling.	I lose control.	I worship.	I eat a snack.	I yell.

65

LOSE IT
for
LIFE
PART 1

If you react to stress with a greatly increased appetite, you may be experiencing higher than normal cortisol levels.

How effective are your typical responses to stress?

_____

_____

Learning a New Way of *Life*

When life gets stressful, our bodies naturally release a hormone called cortisol. During times of ongoing stress, cortisol levels can remain elevated. Since this hormone provides energy for our bodies, it stimulates appetite, making us susceptible to weight gain—especially in the midsection or abdominal area. Pamela Peeke, a former senior scientist at the National Institutes of Health in Bethesda, Maryland, has concluded that three factors affect central fat in women: a poor lifestyle, declining levels of the hormone estrogen, and chronic stress.[5]

What spiritual truths can we apply to these biological realities?

_____

_____

Read Deuteronomy 20:1–4. What "secret" did Moses give the people of Israel as a way to overcome the stress of facing an overwhelming task?

_____

_____

_____

Spend some time reading and pondering Psalm 18. What did David do when facing a heap of trouble from a host of enemies?

_____

_____

_____

What does 1 Peter 5:7 say to those in trouble? How exactly does a person "do" this?

_____

_____

Losing It for *Life*

Because stress is something everyone experiences, we would be wise to learn effective ways to manage or reduce it.

Consider: Some strains and pressures and trials are beyond our control. Facing financial stress because your company suddenly decided to eliminate 2,000 jobs is one thing. Facing financial stress because your credit card spending is wildly out of control is a whole different matter. What could you start doing (or stop doing) today that would make your life less stressful?

_____

_____

LOSE IT
for
LIFE
P A R T   1

We'll end this lesson with five questions designed to help you think about your response to stress in terms of self-care.

What are your most effective ways of relaxing? (Note: Leisure pursuits, hobbies, and so forth keep stress from building up and provide an avenue for releasing tension.)

_____

_____

Relaxing should be a regular, practiced part of your life.

What current exercise routine do you follow? (Note: Exercise can reduce muscle tension and frustration in addition to providing a host of medical helps.)

_____

_____

What is your diet like? Are you eating sensibly? (Note: Our bodies need good healthy foods that provide certain vitamins and minerals.)

_____

_____

Inadequate sleep results in higher cortisol levels, which causes your run-down body to crave carbohydrates and foods high in calories and fat.

How well are you managing your time? (Note: Having healthy priorities and realistic goals can be a great stress-reducer.)

_____

_____

How much and how well are you sleeping? (Note: It is important to go to bed at a regular time and get into a sleep routine.)

_____

_____

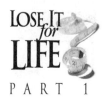

PART 1

DAY 3:
Confronting Reality

After realizing we need to change and deciding that—by the grace of God—we will do so, the next step is taking a realistic, unblinking self-assessment. That's the focus of this lesson.

Looking at Your *Life*

The more you have to lose, the longer it takes. Don't expect to go from 300 pounds to 180 overnight.

How tall are you? And how much did you weigh the last time you stepped on the scales?

_____

_____

How much did you weigh when you graduated from high school or turned 18?

_____

_____

What's the most you've ever weighed? The least (as an adult)?

_____

_____

What size clothes do you wear?

Men	**Women**
Shirt:	Blouse: _____
Knit: _____	
Dress: _____	
Pants:	Pants: _____
Waist: _____	
Inseam: _____	Dress: _____
Suit: _____	

What do you usually do when you pass a large mirror in the hall, or somewhere else? Why?

_____

_____

Learning a New Way of *Life*

You've probably heard the following observations:

- "The unexamined life is not worth living."
- "You cannot possibly get to where you need to be until you first know where you are."
- "Know thyself."
- "If you want to change the world, start by looking in the mirror."

What other sage advice can you recall that urges people to live with healthy self-awareness?

_____

_____

_____

In 2 Corinthians 13:5 the apostle Paul says, "Examine yourselves." In the context of that passage, he is speaking specifically of spiritual assessment. How and why is this a good principle and practice for all of life?

_____

_____

_____

When we are overweight or obese, the last thing we want to do is confront the reality of our size and what it is doing to our body, our health.

Proverbs 27:12 says: "The prudent see danger and take refuge, but the simple keep going and suffer for it." What are the implications of this verse for an overweight person with unhealthy eating and exercise habits?

_____

_____

_____

Why do you think so many people are reluctant to develop the habits of regularly taking stock of their lives or conducting a personal inventory? Why do we resist so strongly the practices that could end up enhancing or even saving our lives?

_____

_____

_____

Losing It for *Life*

Many overweight people avoid taking a good, hard, honest look at their physical bodies. Most look in the mirror only from their necks up. They fix their hair, do their make-up, and put on a happy face. When we are overweight, looking at the entire body is painful and depressing. Taking a full-length view, however, keeps reality in front of us and can be used as incentive to make changes.

In the LIFL book, the authors ask you to stand fully unclothed in front of a full-length mirror, and "slowly scan your entire body." What kinds of feelings does this challenge evoke within you? Put words to your emotions.

_____

_____

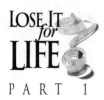

PART 1

Want to take a tremendous step of faith? Follow their counsel. Get the facts. Face reality. Do it. Go ahead. Turn on all the lights so that nothing is hidden, so that the truth is vividly clear for you to see. Afterwards, pull out your pictures or photo album and, with God's help, study yourself objectively. Next, go step on the scales and see exactly where you are. Record your thoughts here:

_____

_____

Begin by setting your weight loss goal at 1 0 percent of your current weight. You can lose weight just by eating 100 calories less a day than you need.

Are we trying to be cruel? No! The goal is to be in touch with the reality of your size and weight. We want you to think about your extra weight and the negative health impact it is having on you. Believe it or not, you can use this to motivate lifestyle changes, not degrade yourself.

Years ago, a popular magazine published a cartoon showing a small group of Chinese individuals standing in the midst of a vast landscape. The caption read, "Well, we have a heck of a wall to build. I suggest we get started."

Funny—in a profound way. What a great reminder that every amazing accomplishment once was nothing but a mere idea, a dream. Yet with a clear plan and lots of hard work and diligence, dreams can and do become reality.

Do this simple exercise. Borrow a child's backpack and fill it up with heavy objects (10–20 pounds worth). Strap it on and do housework or yardwork or walk—for thirty minutes. How do you feel after lugging around this small bit of extra weight?

_____

_____

_____

Now, imagine how much more energy you would have and how much better you would feel if you lost those 20 or 80 or 200 extra pounds of fat you're now carrying!

DAY 4:
Let's Get Physical

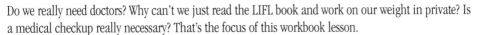

Do we really need doctors? Why can't we just read the LIFL book and work on our weight in private? Is a medical checkup really necessary? That's the focus of this workbook lesson.

Looking at Your *Life*

In your struggle with weight, who is your most sympathetic and understanding ally? Who is your "drill sergeant" (the person who pushes you and tries to motivate you to success)?

_____

_____

_____

A comprehensive physical examination conducted by a competent physician is often necessary to obtain an accurate picture of your health.

Write about your experiences with the medical profession (doctor visits, hospital stays, and so forth.) Do you have positive memories or negative thoughts when you think about your lifetime healthcare history? Why?

_____

_____

_____

_____

Describe your personal physician. What is he or she like? What qualities do you like and admire? What qualities/traits do you wish he or she had?

_____

_____

_____

Learning a New Way of *Life*

Proverbs 15:22 says, "Plans fail for lack of counsel, but with many advisers they succeed."

Write about a time when you embarked upon an ambitious project (for example, a home improvement project, a craft project, and so forth.) without first gathering all the facts or getting the necessary information. What happened? What did you learn?

_____

_____

_____

LOSE IT
for
LIFE

PART 1

In what areas of your life are you typically quick to seek counsel or consult experts? In what areas are you reluctant to ask more knowledgeable heads for help? Why do you think?

_____

_____

_____

A good physician will monitor your medical conditions, support your efforts to make changes, and encourage a holistic approach.

Consider these nuggets from the book of Proverbs that speak about "war":

"Make plans by seeking advice; if you wage war, obtain guidance" (20:18).
"For waging war you need guidance, and for victory many advisers" (24:6).

What do these verses suggest about our own perpetual "war" against fat and obesity? About the need for plans, and guidance, and getting wise advice?

_____

_____

_____

_____

President Coolidge observed, "I not only use all the brains I have, but all I can borrow." What is the value of seeking out expert, professional, medical help when we're not actually sick? Personally, how could you benefit from consulting with a good doctor? List the upside of such a decision.

_____

_____

_____

Losing It for *Life*

When is the last time you had a thorough physical? If it's been a long while, list the specific reasons why you hesitate to have a regular checkup.

_____

_____

_____

_____

In the LIFL book, Dr. Linda described a plaque hanging on her doctor's wall that says: "Let a doctor be called as a healer, not the health care provider. Let the patient be treated as the healed, not the health care consumer. . . . Medicine is not a commercial business but a professional practice based strongly on a doctor-patient relationship of compassion, understanding and respect."[6]

How might your experience be different if you were under the care of such a doctor?

_____

_____

_____

What, realistically, can a physician do for his or her patients? What unrealistic expectations do patients sometimes put upon their doctors?

_____

_____

_____

Unfortunately, we hear too many stories in which doctors simply hand their patients 1200-calorie diets and tell them to lose weight. If this worked, people would be able to follow this advice and drop weight. In our experience, this strategy only compounds feelings of failure. If your physician is insensitive regarding your weight, change doctors and tell your health care company why you are doing so.

We all but guarantee that someone in your immediate network of acquaintances will know a good doctor or be able to point you to someone who does. If you don't currently have one, make it your goal to find a physician who is compassionate and sensitive to overweight people.

Brainstorm some ways you will begin this process.

_____

_____

_____

LOSE IT for LIFE

PART 1

As an overweight person, you already have to contend with ridicule and stigma from the public. You don't need to put up with either from health care providers.

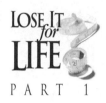

PART 1

Remember that even modest weight loss improves your health.

DAY 5:
The Risks of Obesity

This session will cover some of the most common health risks associated with being overweight. This will not be a comprehensive discussion. We will touch only on main concerns. Our goal is not to scare you or make you fearful but to better inform you. Use this lesson to find the motivation to make healthy changes.

Looking at Your *Life*

In a prior lesson, we asked you for a family medical history. What about your own personal medical condition? What known health issues do you currently face?

_____

_____

What medications do you currently take and for what conditions?

_____

_____

What potential health risks worry you most and why?

_____

_____

Learning a New Way of *Life*

We've quoted this passage before and probably will quote again in this workbook because it speaks directly to the issues we are discussing: "Do you not know that your body is a temple of the Holy Spirit, who is in you, whom you have received from God? You are not your own; you were bought at a price. Therefore honor God with your body" (1 Corinthians 6:19–20).

What are the implications of this truth? What does it say to the person who simply lets himself or herself go?

_____

_____

Proverbs 6:6–11 presents an interesting passage about ants—how they wisely work now so as to have a better future:

> *"Go to the ant, you sluggard; consider its ways and be wise! It has no commander, no overseer or ruler, yet it stores its provisions in summer and gathers its food at harvest.*

How long will you lie there, you sluggard? When will you get up from your sleep? A little sleep, a little slumber, a little folding of the hands to rest—and poverty will come on you like a bandit and scarcity like an armed man."

The point seems to be that the lazy refusal to lift a finger now can lead to big trouble later. How does this principle apply to the whole subject of weight loss and health?

_____

_____

_____

Read Luke 12:16–21. While this parable most pointedly addresses a person's failure to care for his or her spiritual life, it more broadly highlights the foolishness of living a shortsighted life. How does this kind of narrow thinking (living only for the moment) often spill over into the way we care for (or fail to care for) our bodies?

_____

_____

_____

"Dear friend, I pray that you may enjoy good health and that all may go well with you, even as your soul is getting along well" *(3 John 2).*

Losing It for *Life*

Overweight people are foolish to ignore physical warning signs and the findings of modern science. We need to live in the reality that extra weight puts us more at risk for certain health problems. Let's look at the most common health risks of being overweight.

Type 2 Diabetes
(Also referred to as adult onset or non-insulin dependent diabetes; a disease in which blood sugar levels are above normal.)

Did you know . . . ?

- Type 2 diabetes can cause early death, heart disease, kidney disease, stroke, and blindness.
- 80 percent of people with this disease are overweight.[7]
- Losing weight and exercising can lower your risk for Type 2 diabetes.

Heart Disease and Stroke
(Caused when your heart and circulation or blood flow does not operate normally.)

Did you know . . . ?

- Heart disease is the leading cause of death in the United States.[8]
- Strokes are the third leading cause of death in the United States.[9]
- Losing just 5 to 15 percent of your weight can lower your risk for both health problems.

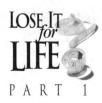

PART 1

Are you anxious? Don't be. Losing as little as 5 percent of your body weight helps. Remember to lose weight slowly and safely.

Cancer

(Occurs when cells in one part of the body grow abnormally or out of control.)

Did you know . . . ?

- When you are overweight, your risk of developing certain types of cancers increases.
- Eating healthy foods and being physically active may lower your risk for cancer.

Sleep Apnea

(When a person stops breathing for short periods during the night.)

Did you know . . . ?

- This condition is more prevalent for people who are overweight.
- Fat stored in the neck area can make the airway for breathing smaller.
- Weight loss improves this condition because it decreases the neck size and inflammation.[10]

Osteoarthritis

(A joint disorder in which the tissues that protect joint bones and cartilage wear away.)

Did you know . . . ?

- The more weight you carry, the more pressure you put on your joints and cartilage.
- Excess weight increases joint inflammation, which increase risk for osteoarthritis.

Gallbladder Disease

Did you know . . . ?

- Overweight people produce more cholesterol, which puts strain on the gallbladder.
- Being overweight means your gallbladder could be enlarged and not work efficiently.[11]
- Losing weight too quickly increases one's chance to develop gallstones.

Fatty Liver Disease

(Results from the build up of fat cells in the liver causing injury and inflammation.)

Did you know . . . ?

- FLD can cause cirrhosis (scar tissue in the liver that blocks blood flow) and liver failure.
- Weight loss helps control blood sugars, which helps avoid the build up of fat in the liver. (Avoiding alcohol helps as well.)[12]

What new things did you learn? What fears do you have? What new resolve?

_____

_____

Preparation: Read chapter five of Lose It for Life *before you begin the lessons for Week 5.*

DAY 1:
RISE Above Your Old Habits (Part 1)

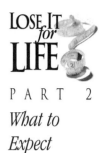

When it comes to eating, popular slogans such as "You are what you eat!" don't help very much. We prefer a more scientific, more practical approach to eating. These lessons will help you decide on an eating plan that's right for you. Our goal is to make healthy lifestyle changes regarding food and eating.

PART 2

What to Expect

Looking at Your *Life*

"Q: How do you eat an elephant? A: One bite at a time." Obviously no one at LIFL wants anyone to eat an elephant or eat *like* an elephant! The point of that familiar maxim is that we accomplish big things by doing little things over and over.

What projects have you completed by chipping away and faithfully plodding ahead?

_____

_____

If you have poor eating habits, changing only one of them can have a dramatic impact.

How are you doing with regard to keeping your food journal? What's the experience been like? In what ways has this habit begun to change your mindset about food and eating?

_____

_____

Skim your journal and note the kinds of foods you eat in a typical day (pick a day from the last couple of weeks). Do certain foods seem to keep "finding their way into your mouth" at certain times of the day? What type of foods and at what times? What's going on here?

_____

_____

The authors make the point that even small changes in amount (one cookie a day instead of three) and small substitutions in the types of food we eat (an apple instead of a Twinkie®) can add up over time to big changes. Have you been able to make small changes like this? Record your thoughts here.

_____

_____

What have you decided about making meal plans? Of the two plans suggested in the *Lose It for Life* book ("The Smart Low Carb Weight Loss Plan" and "The Walker's Weight Loss Plan"), which one is a better fit for you? Why?

_____

_____

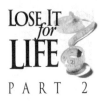

LOSE IT for LIFE

PART 2

Learning a New Way of *Life*

LIFL is more comprehensive than a mere diet; it involves lifestyle changes. As we explore areas in our lives that need to change, a one-word strategy will help: RISE. This acronym reminds us of four actions that need to become our regular habits: *Reduce, Increase, Substitute,* and *Eliminate.* The RISE formula embodies our overall strategy for success and we will apply it to each area of needed change.

If you doubt your ability to succeed in this, spend a few minutes pondering these Bible passages that speak of God's power. Jot down your thoughts and observations after each passage.

As we focus on the acronym RISE, it's helpful to remember that we serve a risen Savior. Not even death could stop Jesus—a fact that should fill us with great hope.

- "I pray also that the eyes of your heart may be enlightened in order that you may know . . . his incomparably great power for us who believe. That power is like the working of his mighty strength, which he exerted in Christ when he raised him from the dead and seated him at his right hand in the heavenly realms" (Ephesians 1:18–20).

  _____

  _____

- "I pray that out of his glorious riches he may strengthen you with power through his Spirit in your inner being" (Ephesians 3:16).

  _____

  _____

- "His divine power has given us everything we need for life and godliness through our knowledge of him who called us by his own glory and goodness" (2 Peter 1:3).

  _____

  _____

What do these verses tell you about God? About his love and care for you? If God is "able"—if he is "for us"—then what should we expect as we endeavor to change by his power?

_____

_____

When have you seen or experienced the power of God?

_____

_____

Losing It for *Life*

Let's begin applying the RISE strategy to our food choices and eating habits by taking a closer look at foods we need to reduce and foods we ought to increase.

Foods to Reduce

There are exceptions, but generally it is wise to cut back on white foods—white sugar, white flour, white rice, potatoes, etc. How much a part of your diet are these foods?

_____

_____

_____

_____

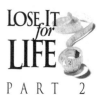

LOSE IT for LIFE

PART 2

"People with a genetic predisposition for addiction can become overly dependent on sugar, particularly if they periodically stop eating and then binge." (Dr. Bart Hoebel)

Take this True/False test about sugar.

T or F?

_____ 1. Too much sugar turns to fat!

_____ 2. Our bodies need sugar to function.

_____ 3. Most carbohydrates contain sugar.

_____ 4. Sugar exists in different forms, some easier to digest than others.

_____ 5. Your body takes the sugar from carbohydrates and converts it to fuel that is either burned or stored. When it is stored, it's called "body fat." The more fuel stored, the more body fat you have!

_____ 6. You can eat as much low-fat stuff as you want without gaining weight.

_____ 7. A candy bar or bag of chips can actually stimulate your hunger by raising your blood sugar levels too quickly.

_____ 8. The so-called "glycemic index" measures the movement of glaciers in northern Canada.

_____ 9. When you significantly reduce or even eliminate high glycemic foods, you will increase your chances to lose weight.

_____ 10. Some research suggests that sugar *may* be addictive.

*[Answers: **1.** True; **2.** True; **3.** False (All carbohydrates contain sugar); **4.** True; **5.** True; **6.** False (Many low-fat foods are high in carbs, which—if not burned—end up stored as fat); **7.** True; **8.** False (The glycemic index measures carbohydrates in food on a scale from 0-100 according to the amount your blood sugar rises after eating it). **9.** True; **10.** True (New studies, mostly with animal subjects, show that overeating sweets may share some characteristics with serious addictions.[1])*

In Appendix C in the *Lose It for Life* book you'll find a glycemic index for a number of foods. Look it over. Which high-glycemic foods are a regular part of your diet?

_____

_____

_____

_____

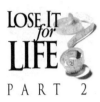

Write about your own relationship with sugar. How about chocolate? Are you a chocoholic? What are some practical, proven ways a person can resist these kinds of high glycemic foods?

_____

_____

Foods to Increase

Fiber is a hugely important part of a healthy eating life-plan. Fiber is that indigestible portion of plant food, found mostly in fresh fruits, vegetables, whole grains, and legumes. Fiber can help us lose weight by slowing down the absorption of sugar and our digestive process, thus decreasing our appetite. Since we can't digest fiber, its bulk gives us a full feeling, which can help us eat less.

What are your favorite foods that are rich in fiber?

_____

_____

Your body automatically warms up cold liquids in order to maintain its internal temperature. Drinking eight glasses of ice water a day burns about 60 calories.[2]

The authors suggest this plan: "Drink 12 ounces of water when you first wake up, 12 ounces before lunch, 12 ounces after lunch, 12 ounces right before dinner, and 12 ounces after dinner."

Does this water plan seem doable for you? Why or why not?

_____

_____

There is good news when it comes to including dairy in your diet. Hard cheeses, yogurt, and milk appear to speed up our metabolisms. Calcium in the blood signals fat cells to stop storing fat and burn it.[3] Including four dairy servings a day is a good idea for weight loss and for building strong bones.

How much dairy product do you eat? What kinds and how often?

_____

_____

Specifically, what foods are you going to reduce? Which ones do you intend to increase?

_____

_____

DAY 2:
RISE Above Your Old Habits (Part 2)

Let's continue the RISE process. We've looked at foods we need to *reduce* and others we need to *increase*. In this session, we'll explore the foods we need to *substitute* and *eliminate* altogether.

Looking at Your *Life*

What are your "guiltiest pleasures" when it comes to eating?

_____

_____

_____

What foods or dishes hold a special place in your heart and mind? Why do you think those items are so enticing to you?

_____

_____

_____

What healthy foods and snacks do you enjoy—that taste good to you?

_____

_____

_____

Increase your consumption of vegetables, lean meats, and fruits low in carbohydrates and high in fiber. Select at least one fruit or vegetable each day.

Learning a New Way of *Life*

Check out the following Bible verses that speak about food and eating.

Then God said, "I give you every seed-bearing plant on the face of the whole earth and every tree that has fruit with seed in it. They will be yours for food" (Genesis 1:29).

Everything that lives and moves will be food for you. Just as I gave you the green plants, I now give you everything (Genesis 9:3).

He makes grass grow for the cattle, and plants for man to cultivate—bringing forth food from the earth (Psalm 104:14).

So whether you eat or drink or whatever you do, do it all for the glory of God (1 Corinthians 10:31).

LOSE IT for LIFE

PART 2

What general conclusions can you draw from these passages about God? About what we can and should eat? About *how* we should eat?

_____

_____

_____

"God ... richly provides us with every-thing for our enjoyment" *(1 Timothy 6:17).*

It's important to remember that LIFL is not a diet. It's a way of life. It's remembering that God is good and that His gifts are good. The key is moderation, not gorging ourselves, and not using food to fill needs it was never intended to fill.

Many, if not most diets absolutely *forbid* certain kinds of food. The LIFL program maintains that no foods are "off-limits." What are the positive benefits of this philosophical difference? What are the potential dangers?

_____

_____

_____

How are you changing as a result of reading, thinking, and applying the LIFL plan?

_____

_____

Losing It for *Life*

LIFL urges us to *reduce* our intake of certain foods and to *increase* our consumption of others. The plan also suggests certain things to substitute or eliminate altogether.

Foods to Substitute

Obviously it is wise to substitute high-fat foods that contain little nutritional value with low-fat healthy foods.

Using your food journal as a guide, list some substitutions you could and should make that would lead to a healthier you.

_____

_____

_____

It is also wise to substitute high glycemic foods with low ones. Some examples: eating fruit-flavored yogurt instead of a glazed doughnut, vegetables and dip instead of potato chips and dip, a bean burrito instead of a beef burrito, and so forth.

Again, look at the record of your recent eating habits. Using Appendix C of the *Lose It for Life* book, suggest at least five food substitutions you could begin making regularly, that—over time—would result in a big difference.

_____

_____

_____

LOSE IT
for
LIFE
PART 2

The authors urge us to try new foods, noting that some food items we never liked as children we would enjoy now. List personal examples of this.

Foods I Hated When I Was Younger   When I Learned to Like Them

_____

_____

_____

_____

Now list some other not-so-favorite foods (low in fat and low on the glycemic index) that you will agree to go back and try again.

_____

_____

_____

Foods to Eliminate

We've seen that fats and proteins slow down sugar absorption. Yet we've also noted that not all fats are the same. One type of fat is downright dangerous, so we want to eliminate it as much as possible. The fat to avoid at all costs is *trans fatty acid,* also called "trans fat."

Take a short True/False quiz and see how much you remember from the LIFL book about trans fat.

_____ 1. Trans fatty acid is created when our diets include too much beef and too many carbonated drinks.

_____ 2. Adding trans fat to a food increases its shelf life and often gives it a good flavor.

_____ 3. Too much trans fat can lead to obesity, a weakened immune system, diabetes, coronary heart disease, muscle loss, increased cancer risk, and global warming.

_____ 4. About 40 percent of the food on grocery store shelves contains partially hydrogenated vegetable oils, which contain trans fatty acid.

_____ 5. The way to tell how much trans fat a food item has is to look at the label. If you see the words "hydrogenated" or "partially hydrogenated" anywhere near the top of the ingredients list, the food is high in trans fat.

_____ 6. Typically, organic foods have more trans fat than foods processed in modern factories.

PART 2

There is a distant cousin of trans fat called CLA (conjugated linoleic acid) that naturally occurs in dairy and beef. New studies show that CLA may actually be helpful in fighting off the very thing its cousin brings about. [5]

*[Answers: **1.** False ("Trans fat" is a man-made substance produced when hydrogen is bubbled through oil to produce a margarine that doesn't melt at room temperature); **2.** True [4]; **3.** False (Everything but the global warming part); **4.** True; **5.** True; **6.** False (The truth is just the opposite; natural foods are healthier than processed ones.)]*

Where do you see a lot of trans fats in your diet? What particular foods?

_____

_____

_____

Take a field trip to your pantry. List the items you find there that are high in trans fatty acid.

_____

_____

_____

Some practical tips for eliminating the scourge of trans fat: switch to milk instead of nondairy creamer in your coffee, use oil or sesame oil or butter flavored spray instead of margarines, and choose baked chips over fried, as ways to cut down or eliminate trans fat.

What's the most powerful or helpful thing you've learned in this lesson? Why?

_____

_____

_____

DAY 3:
What's on the Menu?

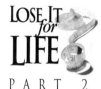

LOSE IT
for
LIFE

PART 2

We all *have* to eat. We all *want* to eat. We have a myriad of choices, but not all choices are wise ones. Our goal in this lesson is to take a look at menus—to begin to formulate a personalized eating plan that is both nutritious and delicious; a plan that will help us drop extra weight and keep it off for life.

Looking at Your *Life*

Just for fun, think back to school lunches. What do you remember? Did you eat in the cafeteria or bring your lunch? Write a few memories in the space below.

_____

_____

Choose fruits and vegetables with vivid colors. You can't go wrong by choosing these "nutrient powerhouses."

Try to list 10 foods that taste good and are good for you. Which ones are part of your regular diet?

_____

_____

_____

We can fall into certain eating patterns in which we tend to eat the same dishes time and time again. Consider your own eating habits. In a typical month, what are the meals you eat, what are the snacks you seek out, and what restaurants do you dine in? In other words, what foods comprise the bulk of your personal menu?

Top Ten Meals (Home-cooked)   How Many Times Eaten Per Month

_____   _____

_____   _____

_____   _____

_____   _____

_____   _____

Top Ten Snacks   How Many Times Eaten Per Month

_____   _____

_____   _____

_____   _____

_____   _____

_____   _____

LOSE IT
for
LIFE
PART 2

Top Ten Meals (Restaurant)   How Many Times Eaten Per Month

_____

_____

_____

_____

_____

"So do not worry, saying, 'What shall we eat?' or 'What shall we drink?' or 'What shall we wear?' . . . your heavenly Father knows that you need them" (Matthew 6:31–32).

Based on what you've learned thus far, what problems do you see with your existing eating habits?

_____

_____

Learning a New Way of *Life*

Paul has an interesting paragraph in his letter to the Philippian Christians. He wrote:

> *"Join with others in following my example, brothers, and take note of those who live according to the pattern we gave you. For, as I have often told you before and now say again even with tears, many live as enemies of the cross of Christ. Their destiny is destruction, their god is their stomach, and their glory is in their shame. Their mind is on earthly things. But our citizenship is in heaven. And we eagerly await a Savior from there, the Lord Jesus Christ, who, by the power that enables him to bring everything under his control, will transform our lowly bodies so that they will be like his glorious body" (Philippians 3:17–21).*

Notice the phrase "their god is their stomach." In other words, these worldly people are slaves to their own sensual appetites and physical desires. Whatever urges they sense within, they immediately follow and seek to satisfy. Paul contrasts this kind of immediate gratification mindset and lifestyle with believers who have an eternal perspective.

In what ways can the desire for food become all-consuming—like a "god"?

_____

_____

_____

What's involved in making the switch between "living to eat" and "eating to live"?

_____

_____

_____

Read and ponder Matthew 6:25–34. How do these words of Christ provide new perspective on life (including the role of food)?

_____

_____

Losing It for *Life*

The LIFL book contains all kinds of practical ideas for menu development. Which ones strike your fancy? Jot down the tips and suggestions that you'd like to try.

_____

_____

Chapter five of *Lose It for Life* helps you calculate your current calorie intake and activity level. Based on the chart in the book, are you sedentary, active, or very active? How many calories do you estimate that you burn daily?

_____

_____

Using the formulas and following the directions in the book, what calorie level intake do you need in order to lose a pound or two a week?

_____

_____

Look at the five-day meal plan in Appendix D in *Lose It for Life.* This menu is based upon 125 grams of carbs a day. What do you like about this plan?

_____

_____

"The Walker's Weight Loss Plan" is featured in Appendix D. Take a few minutes to study the week-long menu provided there. What's your assessment? How could this work for you?

_____

_____

Reduce your current calorie intake by 500 to 1,000 calories a day. This will lead to safe, effective weight loss of 1 to 2 pounds per week.

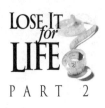

DAY 4:
Common Sense for Uncommon Weight Control

Some people get so immersed in calories and carbs, and in the science of fats and fitness, that they lose sight of simple, basic truths. The goal of this lesson is to remember some common sense practices that can lead to uncommon success in losing it for life.

Looking at Your *Life*

"Wisdom is supreme; therefore get wisdom. Though it cost all you have, get under-standing" (Proverbs 4:7).

A few years ago, a best-selling book offered everyday wisdom gleaned from the lives of regular folks. For example, "I've learned it's possible to do something in a moment that you'll regret for a lifetime." Or "I've learned that when all is said and done, more things are said than done."

Following that same format, what are some lessons you've learned about food and eating in your lifetime. (EX: "I've learned that I should *never* go grocery shopping when I'm hungry!")

_____

_____

_____

What's been the most helpful advice or suggestion you've received so far in your participation in the Lose It For Life system? Why?

_____

_____

_____

In what specific ways do your LIFL comrades encourage you to keep persevering?

_____

_____

_____

What about your family and friends? What's been their attitude as you have embarked on this new weight-loss/weight management life plan?

_____

_____

_____

Have you been to the LIFL website? If not, take some time right now, log on to the World Wide Web, and surf your way over to **www.loseitforlife.com**. You'll find many interesting features and articles.

Learning a New Way of *Life*

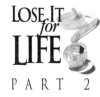

Just for fun, take this food quiz and test your knowledge of eating habits in Bible times. Match the following questions with the correct answers.

_____ 1. What strange snack did Samson eat?

_____ 2. What was John the Baptist's weird diet?

_____ 3. What unusual food had the appearance of coriander seed?

_____ 4. What did the Hebrews eat in Egypt?

_____ 5. What was on King Solomon's daily menu?

_____ 6. What food did Jacob use to get his brother's birthright?

_____ 7. What meal did Jacob cook to steal his father's blessing?

_____ 8. What foods did the Mosaic Law forbid the Jews to eat?

_____ 9. What foods were part of the Passover Meal?

_____ 10. What food "gift" did the sons of Jacob present to Joseph when they arrived in Egypt to buy grain?

a. Camels, hares, snakes, ostrich, locusts (see Leviticus 11)

b. Cooked goat (see Genesis 27:14–18)

c. Fish, cucumbers, melons, leeks, onions and garlic (see Numbers 11:5)

d. Locusts and honey (see Matthew 3:4)

e. Bread, beef, lamb, goat, deer, gazelle, roebuck and choice fowl (see 1 Kings 4:22–23)

f. Roasted lamb, unleavened bread, bitter herbs (see Exodus 12:1–10)

g. Bread and lentil ("red") stew (see Genesis 25:27–34)

h. Honey, out of a lion's carcass (see Judges 14:5–9)

i. Almonds (see Genesis 43:11)

j. Manna (see Exodus 16:31)

*(Answers: **1.** h; **2.** d; **3.** j; **4.** c; **5.** e; **6.** g; **7.** b; **8.** a; **9.** f; **10.** i)*

Read Jesus' comments in John 4:32–34. What do you think he meant? In what way is doing God's will "food"?

_____

_____

_____

_____

LOSE IT
for
LIFE
PART 2

What are the implications of this for your life?

_____

_____

_____

_____

We can't tell you how many people think losing weight is about skipping breakfast. They couldn't be more wrong!

Losing It for *Life*

What reasons are given in the LIFL book for eating breakfast? What's your own experience? How has skipping breakfast helped or hurt you?

_____

_____

_____

Why is weighing one's self regularly a good practice to develop?

_____

_____

_____

Keeping a daily account of your weight will give you the feedback you need to cut back or maintain your weight.

What might happen if you downsize your portions? For example, eat two cookies instead of three, an 8 oz. steak instead of a 12 oz. steak, leave some food on your plate when dining out. If you did this consistently for six months, what might happen? How would it make a difference?

_____

_____

_____

If you increased your intake of foods that are lower in calories and higher in density, such as veggies and low-cal soups, what can result?

_____

_____

_____

_____

The authors suggest eating more often. "If you eat six mini meals a day, you don't have to pack in the food in order to 'make it' until the next meal four hours later. Instead, eat smaller meals every two hours. In fact, research supports the idea that people who eat smaller, frequent meals are thinner and healthier."[6]

What are your thoughts about mini meals? Have you tried this? With what results?

_____

_____

_____

Lose It
for
LIFE

They also recommend a regular eating routine, because the more variety you have to choose from, the greater the likelihood of overeating. In what ways have you experienced this fact personally?

_____

_____

_____

Why is it a bad idea to go to a big event hungry?

_____

_____

_____

When you are trying to lose weight, don't cook or bake or buy rich, fatty foods you will be tempted to eat.

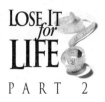

PART 2

DAY 5:
Handling Dangerous (Food) Situations

We've been looking at the practical things about eating and reminding ourselves of some common food traps and some common sense solutions. Let's continue in that vein, focusing in this short lesson on how to create an overall safer eating environment.

It's very important to create an eating atmosphere that is free of anxiety. Mealtime should be enjoyable and relaxing.

Looking at Your *Life*

Most of us know ourselves well enough to know our tendencies. In what situations are you most inclined to overeat? Why?

_____

_____

_____

When was the last time you ate so much you felt physically ill?

_____

_____

_____

When was the last time you said no to a tantalizing food temptation? How did you manage to do it? How did you feel afterwards?

_____

_____

_____

Describe meal times around your house. What's the mood like—before, during, and after? What goes on in your own heart? Why?

_____

_____

_____

_____

Learning a New Way of *Life*

If while driving down the highway, you suddenly encountered a series of warning signs (for example, "Bridge out ahead" or "Left lane closed"), you would slow down, right? You'd become more aware, more careful.

LOSE IT
for
LIFE

P A R T   2

Proverbs 22:3 says, "A prudent man sees danger and takes refuge, but the simple keep going and suffer for it." This verse suggests a very wise principle: Be on the lookout, be smart. Don't make foolish avoidable decisions that lead to unnecessary grief.

Let's apply that to eating. What are the warning signs for you that you might be entering a "dangerous food zone"?

_____

_____

_____

Proverbs 23:2–3 (THE MESSAGE) states, "Don't gobble your food, don't talk with your mouth full. And don't stuff yourself; bridle your appetite." Your reaction?

_____

_____

_____

You can create an eating atmosphere that is soothing and peaceful . . . and conducive to losing weight and keeping it off.

Ponder this amazing verse for a few minutes: "No temptation has seized you except what is common to man. And God is faithful; he will not let you be tempted beyond what you can bear. But when you are tempted, he will also provide a way out so that you can stand up under it" (1 Corinthians 10:13).

What does this passage promise?

_____

_____

_____

What are some "ways out" for us when we find ourselves in the midst of tempting sumptuous food situations?

_____

_____

_____

What are the implications of this verse for us as we strive to settle into a healthier lifestyle of eating right and exercising consistently?

_____

_____

_____

Losing It for *Life*

LOSE IT for LIFE

PART 2

What are some reasons that soft music, candles, and positive conversation can help us develop a new attitude about eating?

_____

_____

Read through the following list of eating habits. Why do you think each of these can be "dangerous" habits sometimes?

Eating too hurriedly

_____

Eating at irregular times

_____

Eating in front of the TV

_____

Eating in the car

_____

Eating while reading

_____

Eating while standing

_____

Eating while you cook

_____

Eating at other places than the dining table or breakfast bar

_____

Which of those habits are you guilty of?

_____

_____

_____

Write a comment or two about each of the following—specifically why they are *wise* habits.
  Chewing food slowly

_____

  Putting your fork down between bites

_____

  Drinking water with your meal

_____

  Eating off a smaller plate

_____

  Ridding your house of tempting high fat foods

_____

  Wrapping leftovers in foil rather than plastic wrap

_____

  Putting leftovers away, out of sight

_____

  Changing the channel or turning the page when you see a food out on TV or in a magazine

_____

  Eating in front of others

_____

Which three positive habits can you (*will* you) implement today?

_____

_____

Go back and review the authors' suggestions for dining out, found in chapter five of the book. Of the
ten tips they give, which two or three will you put into effect the next time you go out to eat?

_____

_____

_____

LOSE IT
for
LIFE

PART 2

Choose an eating plan and foods that will improve your energy and health. Even just a few changes, over time, will produce a healthier, thinner you.

Preparation: Read chapter six of Lose It for Life *before you begin the lessons for Week 6.*

DAY 1:
Exercise 101—Do We Have To?

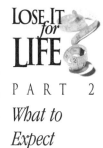

PART 2
What to Expect

You've heard the saying, "Move it or lose it!" We'd like to alter that a bit to say, "Move it *and* lose it." The more you move your body, the more calories you'll burn and the more fat you'll lose. Exercise may never turn you into an Olympian, but it *is* a huge part of shedding excess weight and keeping it off. That's our focus in these five sessions.

Looking at Your *Life*

Begin by examining your attitude towards exercise. Check all the statements that are true of you.

_____ I absolutely *detest* the thought of exercise.

_____ It's tough for me to find the time to exercise.

_____ I frankly don't like to sweat.

_____ I have had some negative exercise experiences in my life.

_____ I'd rather chill out on the couch than engage in physical activities.

_____ Give me the elevator over the stairs any day!

_____ I always fail in my commitments to exercise.

_____ Most of my friends and family are sedentary.

_____ I need to lose weight first—then, I'll exercise.

_____ Even a brief walk or small bit of exertion wears me out.

How many check marks do you have? _____

If exercise sounds like torture to you, don't worry! We are convinced you can find physical activities that you really enjoy.

Now, evaluate yourself against this scale:

0–2—Awesome! You are knocking on the door of great success!

3–5—With just a few minor attitude adjustments, you'll be burning some serious calories!

6–10—Time to think long and hard about some serious questions: Do you *really* want to continue living an unhealthy existence of being overweight and tired all the time and living a life that revolves around food? Aren't you hungry for a richer, fuller, happier lifestyle? Wouldn't you rather be "weightless," that is, free from the trap of fat, feeling fit, finding joy in the Lord, not in food)?

Learning a New Way of *Life*

Philippians 4:8 says, "Finally, brothers, whatever is true, whatever is noble, whatever is right, whatever is pure, whatever is lovely, whatever is admirable—if anything is excellent or praiseworthy—think about such things."

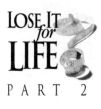

If exercise is good and right for us, how might the verse above apply to our approach to it?

_____

_____

How does *your* thinking need to change regarding exercise?

_____

_____

We've already applied the RISE formula (Reduce, Increase, Substitute, and Eliminate) to eating. Now let's apply it to exercise. Give some specific examples in each of the following:

When it comes to exercise, I need to reduce . . .

_____

_____

When it comes to exercise, I need to increase . . .

_____

_____

When it comes to exercise, I need to substitute . . .

_____

_____

When it comes to exercise, I need to eliminate . . .

_____

_____

Losing It for *Life*

According to the book, is it better to have several short-bursts of exercise daily or longer, once-a-day physical exertions? What's the optimal amount of exercise daily?

_____

_____

What are the implications of this research as you look at your personal schedule?

_____

_____

List some of the *benefits* of exercise cited in the *Lose It for Life* book. Which of these facts surprise you the most? Which of these benefits would you most like to see in your life?

_____

_____

We find time—or *make* time—for the things we value and consider important. How can you adjust your schedule so that you can begin exercising on a regular basis?

_____

_____

What would you say to friends who made the following arguments about exercising?

- "Thanks, but I'm going to lose weight by simply dieting."

_____

_____

- "I walked consistently for two weeks and didn't see any results!"

_____

_____

- "Running around the block? Getting on an exercise bike? Exercise is boring!"

_____

_____

- "I don't have time to exercise!"

_____

_____

- "Nobody will exercise with me, and I just can't do it by myself!"

_____

_____

- "Aerobics? Are you kidding? I get winded if I walk out to the mailbox!"

_____

_____

- "Money's tight right now—I can't afford a health club membership."

_____

_____

LOSE IT
for
LIFE

PART 2

Your attitude towards exercising matters. Consider it as important as the food you put in your mouth. Exercise isn't optional in Lose It For Life.

If you are over 35 and have been inactive for several years, you should consult with a doctor first.

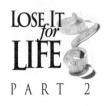

PART 2

DAY 2:
Simple (and Sensible) Strategies

Maybe you haven't exercised in years. Maybe a simple stroll around the block wears you out. Maybe you can't afford a health club membership. Not to worry. Don't let any of that discourage you! You can do this. By God's grace and with common sense and a little effort, you can begin the process of shaping up. That's the focus of this lesson.

Looking at Your *Life*

Think back to when you were a child. What were you favorite activities? What active games did you play? Which ones were you good at?

_____

_____

What organized sports did you play?

_____

_____

What kind of chores and jobs were you assigned around the house?

_____

_____

_____

If nothing were stopping you (money, being overweight, and so forth), what sport or recreational pursuit would you like to participate in? Why?

_____

_____

Circle the following descriptions that apply to you. *"I'm more motivated to exercise . . ."*

First thing in the morning   Midday   Afternoon   After work/Evening

By myself   With others   *Against* others (that is, in competitive situations)

Inside   Outside   At a health club

If the activity is purposeful   If the activity is mindless

If I buy some new video or exercise equipment

If the activity is new   If the activity is something I'm good at

Why is it important to understand yourself, your likes, dislikes, and passions when trying to create an exercise regimen?

_____

_____

Learning a New Way of *Life*

Any worthwhile endeavor takes time, and we have to start *where we are*. Whether you are 25 or 250 pounds overweight, so be it. Your weight is what it is—but not for long. We're going to get you moving. And you're going to learn to like it, because in time you're going to start feeling better and looking better.

"The longest journey begins with the first step." (Chinese proverb)

The laws of physics tell us, "A body at rest tends to remain at rest; a body in motion tends to remain in motion." Why is that worth mentioning here? What's the point?

_____

_____

In the book of Proverbs, a "sluggard" is a person with no discipline or motivation, in short, a foolish failure. He or she is lazy in every way—mentally, spiritually, morally, financially, and so forth. A sluggard takes the path of least resistance. Some descriptive examples:

- "How long will you lie there, you sluggard? When will you get up from your sleep?" (Proverbs 6:9)
- "Lazy hands make a man poor, but diligent hands bring wealth" (Proverbs 10:4).
- "As a door turns on its hinges, so a sluggard turns on his bed. The sluggard buries his hand in the dish; he is too lazy to bring it back to his mouth" (Proverbs 26:14–15).
- "The sluggard craves and gets nothing, but the desires of the diligent are fully satisfied" (Proverbs 13:4).
- "The way of the sluggard is blocked with thorns, but the path of the upright is a highway" (Proverbs 15:19).

What is the overall picture painted here? Do you *like* being around this kind of person? Do you want to *be* a sluggish, aimless individual, existing and not accomplishing anything?

_____

_____

Laziness is often a primary reason we fail to exercise. What other reasons might we have for not engaging in physical activity?

_____

_____

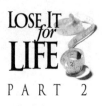

PART 2

Losing It for *Life*

Exercise is much broader than what you do in a health club or something that requires special equipment. In all sorts of ingenious, simple ways, we can move our bodies and burn calories daily. The LIFL book listed some creative examples of this: getting up to change the TV channel instead of using a remote, getting off the bus or subway one stop early and walking the rest of the way, walking around while you talk on the cordless phone, and so forth.

Choose physical activities that mesh well with who you are and what you like to do. You'll be more likely to stick to them.

Think for a few moments about *your* everyday life. Brainstorm 10 ways to avoid becoming an inactive couch potato; to begin moving and speed up the old metabolism.

_____

_____

What sorts of activities would be ideal for a person who likes new things, new physical and/or mental challenges?

_____

_____

What kind of workout regimen would you recommend for a person who gets bored easily or hates too much routine and structure? Why?

_____

_____

If you're an outdoorsy type person, include nature in your exercise routine. Try hiking, biking, nature walking, gardening, lap swimming, or cross-country skiing.

What are the pros and cons of exercising early in the morning? At lunch? In the evening?

_____

_____

What are your conclusions at the end of this lesson?

_____

_____

DAY 3:
Safety Reminders

PART 2

Here's what you *don't* need—deciding to get active only to injure yourself (a pulled muscle, a strained back, and so forth). This puts you in worse shape than before you started to lose it for life! The object of this lesson is to look at some basic safeguards for exercise success.

Looking at Your *Life*

What's your all-time worst exercise or sports injury? What is your "Achilles' heel" (a vulnerable or weak spot) when it comes to physical training?

_____

_____

We've all heard the phrase "no pain, no gain" used in reference to exercise. To what extent is this advice true? When does this sentiment go too far?

_____

_____

Do you grunt or groan involuntarily when you bend over or squat or exert yourself? What does this mean, if anything?

_____

_____

Rank from 1 to 10 these fitness fiascos by their severity *to you* (1 = "earth shattering"; 10 = "no big deal").

_____ Spraining an ankle

_____ Pulling a hamstring

_____ Breaking in new pair running/walking shoes

_____ Tripping and falling off a treadmill in front of a bunch of strangers at a health club

_____ Getting shin splints

_____ Getting athlete's foot

_____ Developing blisters on your feet

_____ Being chased on your bike by a vicious dog

_____ Getting drilled in the "caboose" with a hard-hit racquetball

_____ Dropping some weights on your foot

Don't focus on what you can't do. Don't worry about how others may perceive you. Instead, ask God for courage and then do something.

Whenever you exercise, drink plenty of water before, during, and after exercising to keep your body hydrated.

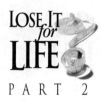

PART 2

Learning a New Way of *Life*

Jeremiah 29:11 says, "For I know the plans I have for you," declares the LORD, "plans to prosper you and not to harm you, plans to give you hope and a future." This verse technically applies to the Old Testament people of God. The prophet Jeremiah spoke it to the Jewish nation just before they experienced judgment at the hands of Babylon. God wanted His people to know that He wasn't finished with them. After a time of exile would come restoration and a glorious future.

What comfort can people of God today draw from this verse? What does it suggest about the character of God, His control of our lives, and His heart for His children?

_____

_____

_____

Given glimpses of the Almighty like this one, how do you know that God wants to see you succeed in your LIFL venture? Why or why not?

_____

_____

_____

Read Philippians 4:6–7 and 1 Peter 5:7. What are these passages about? What relevance do they have as you contemplate (perhaps anxiously) embarking on a more rigorous exercise routine?

_____

_____

_____

If God has knowledge of seemingly trivial facts such as how many hairs we have on our heads (Luke 12:6–7), then what can we conclude about His keeping track of our efforts to burn calories and get in better shape?

_____

_____

_____

Losing It for *Life*

The LIFL book mentions the importance of paying attention to our bodies when we exercise. Five physical warning signs (signals to stop exercising) are given in chapter six. List them here.

_____

_____

Which of those "red flags," if any, have you experienced lately?

_____

_____

_____

LOSE IT
for
LIFE
PART 2

Why is lightweight, loose-fitting clothing important to wear when you exercise?

_____

_____

_____

Exercise helps manage hunger. Research shows that increased exercise increases control over hunger and food intake.[2]

Which of the following do you have and routinely use?

_____ Personal support (an athletic bra for women, athletic supporter for men)

_____ Well-fitting shoes designed for the kind of activity in which you are engaging

_____ A hat for warmth in winter, and sunlight/heat protection in summer

_____ Sunscreen for outdoor activities

_____ Sweat suits that absorb perspiration, removing it from your skin

The authors make the case that exercise really *does* get easier over time. Has this been your experience? Give some examples.

_____

_____

_____

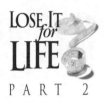

DAY 4:
Getting Started

How tragic that for many people exercise is a hated or dreaded part of life. Moving your body (that is, burning calories, building muscle, losing weight, and so forth) can and should become a joyous and life-enhancing activity. That's our goal. In this session we'll find motivation to get going.

Looking at Your *Life*

Think about your schedule. When are your most convenient or most ideal exercise slots? Why is convenience an important factor in physical fitness success?

_____

_____

What activities do you most enjoy? What "sports" do you truly dislike and why? Why is "having fun" an important part of your exercise success?

_____

_____

Are you the kind of person who likes variety—in your diet, or your clothes, or on vacation? How might a varied exercise regimen help you reach your goals?

_____

_____

An exercise partner can provide accountability and encouragement.

Think about your circle of friends and acquaintances. Which friend(s) do you seek out when you . . .

Want to laugh?

_____

Want to be challenged in your thinking—want a good intellectual exchange?

_____

Want to be encouraged and inspired?

_____

Need some support?

_____

Are looking for wisdom or counsel?

_____

_____

How could you combine some of these friendships with your exercise needs and goals?

_____

_____

_____

Learning a New Way of *Life*

Don't forget Paul's words in 1 Timothy 4:8 (NLT): "Physical exercise has some value, but spiritual exercise is much more important, for it promises a reward in both this life and the next."

What conclusions can we/should we draw from this verse?

_____

_____

What are the limits of physical exercise? In other words what can it do for us and *not* do for us?

_____

_____

_____

What spiritual exercises are part of your daily routine? Why are these disciplines important?

_____

_____

_____

Losing It for *Life*

As you can see, the decision to exercise will take *commitment*. Don't be afraid of that word. You can do this with God's help and the help of others.

Three kinds of exercise are important for all-around fitness. These are listed in chapter six. Do you remember what they are and why each is important? Give some examples of each.

_____

_____

_____

LOSE IT
for
LIFE
PART 2

You may decide you prefer to work-out alone because it's the one place in your schedule you can have peace and quiet.

LOSE IT for LIFE

PART 2

Some people who haven't exercised for many years are put off by the thought of strength training. Maybe it conjures up images of smelly gyms and muscle-bound freaks. What are some strength-training exercises you can do that don't require a set of weights?

_____

_____

_____

If you do not carve out time for your physical, spiritual, and personal needs, you will burn out, bum out, and bail out by acting out.

What muscles in your body are especially weak?

_____

_____

_____

Why is stretching important?

_____

_____

_____

The LIFL book suggests that we put our fitness goals and routine on paper and set some strict boundaries to guard that time. Why is this an important step? Have you done this? If not, stop and do so now.

_____

_____

_____

Why is it important to start slowly with any new exercise routine?

_____

_____

_____

What good purpose can an exercise journal serve?

_____

_____

_____

DAY 5:
Options Galore!

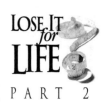

LOSE IT
for
LIFE
PART 2

Aren't you glad to have so many food options? Imagine a life in which we ate gruel—and only gruel—every single day. Thank the Lord for so much variety! In the same way, there are lots of possibilities for exercise. We conclude this week of lessons with a final look at your fitness options, and a few reminders.

Any kind of activity is good, but experts recommend 20–30 minutes of vigorous aerobic activity three or more times a week.

Looking at Your *Life*

Describe your experiences of the following activities when you were a kid. When did you do these activities? How did you feel when you did them?

Riding bike

_____

_____

Skating

_____

_____

Dancing

_____

_____

Hiking

_____

_____

Do you agree that "variety is the spice of life"? Or, are you the kind of person who becomes overwhelmed and/or paralyzed when presented with a broad array of options? Why?

_____

_____

What's a sport or leisure pursuit you've always wanted to try? Why does it intrigue you?

_____

_____

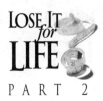

PART 2

Swimming or water aerobics is an excellent way to burn calories and strengthen the heart. The buoyancy of the water helps reduce stress on our joints. Is swimming something you like? If not, what is difficult about it for you?

_____

_____

The key to successful weight control and improved overall health is making physical activity a part of your daily life.

Learning a New Way of *Life*

We humans tend to be superficial, focusing mostly on externals. God looks deeper (see 1 Samuel 16:7). He's more concerned with the condition of our souls.

As you add exercise to your busy schedule, how can you also make sure you maintain a close relationship with God? Any ideas for doing both at once (that is, exercising physically and spiritually)?

_____

_____

If you're a mom or a dad, if you're a church member, if you have a circle of friends, if you have bills to pay, and so forth, you always have a zillion things you could be doing other than exercise. With an endless number of needs around you, you may even feel it's selfish to think of carving out 30–45 minutes a day for yourself (specifically for your own physical and spiritual health and well-being).

What do the following passages say about taking time alone?

Matthew 4:13:

_____

_____

Mark 1:35:

_____

_____

Mark 6:31:

_____

_____

Luke 5:16:

_____

_____

We must take care of ourselves by setting boundaries with our time and energy so we have time for important personal priorities, like eating right and exercising. It is important to decide in advance that your fitness, nutrition, spiritual, and personal time is non-negotiable. You are no good to anyone else if your own body and soul are falling apart.

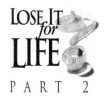

P A R T   2

Losing It for *Life*

Why do the authors suggest that beginners slowly and gradually increase the frequency, intensity, and length of their workouts?

_____

_____

_____

The authors recommend engaging in little bursts of exercise each day. Check the boxes of the ones you think are doable for you.

- ❑ Marching or running in place
- ❑ Kicks
- ❑ Jump rope
- ❑ Waist twists

- ❑ Crossovers
- ❑ Punches
- ❑ Jump squats
- ❑ Jack-in-the-box

If those exercises seem a bit too strenuous, which of the following ones seem more suited to you?
- ❑ Doing standing squats as you blow-dry or curl your hair
- ❑ Pacing or marching in place while you talk on the phone
- ❑ Taking the stairs whenever possible, instead of the elevator
- ❑ Squeezing your buttock muscles as you stand at the stove or fold laundry
- ❑ Doing leg-raises while you watch TV
- ❑ "Zipping in" your abs while you iron
- ❑ Putting on lively music and "dancing" while you mop
- ❑ Using a push mower instead of a riding mower

What other simple, creative ways can you find to get your heart pumping while you are going about mundane tasks?

_____

_____

_____

What are some of the advantages and benefits of *cycling*?

_____

_____

LOSE IT
for
LIFE

PART 2

*Get motivated,
get committed,
get accountable,
and get moving
so you can lose
it for life!*

What are some of the advantages and benefits of *walking*?

_____

_____

_____

What's the difference between *walking* and *hiking*? Which do you prefer and why?

_____

_____

_____

Why are the right shoes such an important part of a walking exercise regimen?

_____

_____

_____

When should a person consult his or her physician before starting a new fitness program?

_____

_____

_____

It's time to get moving! Perhaps exercise will be your biggest challenge. If you are overweight, it hurts both physically and emotionally to move your body. But you can start slow. Take baby steps. Be patient. Remember you're not in a race; you're embarking on a new lifestyle. Give yourself plenty of grace (God does!).

And remember this great truth: "Let us not become weary in doing good, for at the proper time we will reap a harvest if we do not give up" (Galatians 6:9). Technically the verse is speaking about doing good to others, but the deeper principle still holds. Doing right, over time, ultimately results in good results.

Preparation: Read chapter seven of Lose It for Life *before you begin the lessons for Week 7.*

DAY 1:
Emotional Eating

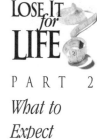

LOSE IT
for
LIFE

P A R T   2

What to Expect

In the next few pages we will look in greater detail at the important and surprisingly large role our emotions often play in our relationship with food. Before you begin, ask God to open your eyes to the truths you need to see, embrace, and live out. Ask him for the courage to make any necessary changes.

Looking at Your *Life*

Chapter seven in *Lose It for Life* begins with some journal entries of a woman named Cathy. What situations in her life do you most relate to, and why?

_____

_____

Do others see you as an *emotional* person? How do you see yourself?

_____

_____

_____

Some people bottle up all their emotions, sweeping them under the proverbial rug. Others go through life absolutely dominated by their changing feelings. What are the problems with each approach?

_____

_____

"I stuffed away sad or emotional times by eating until I was emotionally numb. Now I've stopped medicating with food, and it's incredible to actually 'feel' my emotions— good and bad."—Cathy, a Lose It For Life member

Learning a New Way of *Life*

The unique claim of Christianity is that Almighty God stepped out of eternity into time in the person of Jesus Christ (John 1:1, 14). What a jaw-dropping truth—the Creator entering his own creation, to rescue us (Luke 19:10) and to show us what he is like (John 1:18)!

So what was Jesus like? What did he do? The Gospel writers record matter-of-factly that Jesus possessed and displayed a variety of human emotions:

- He wept (John 11:35).
- He got angry (Mark 3:5).
- He felt distressed and troubled (Mark 14:33).
- He was sorrowful (Matthew 26:37).
- He was joyful (Luke 10:21).
- He (apparently) got exasperated (Luke 9:41).
- He felt weary and tired (John 4:6; Mark 4:38).

LOSE IT
for
LIFE

PART 2

Sometimes we feel as if we'll be swept away by the force of our emotions. But God pledges His comfort, peace, and presence, no matter what.

If the perfect God-man felt all these things, what does that suggest to you about feelings?

_____

_____

_____

_____

It is common for us to assume that good feelings and times are positive and should be pursued, while bad feelings and hard times should be avoided at all costs. Yet the Bible offers a different perspective on the "negative" unpleasant trials of life.

Read Romans 5:1–5. What surprises you about this passage? What are some good things that can come out of unpleasant experiences?

_____

_____

_____

Many people read, memorize, and discuss Romans 8:28. What does this verse suggest about the subject at hand?

_____

_____

_____

Read two or three psalms (try any from Psalms 1–15). What emotions do you see expressed in these ancient Hebrew songs? What conclusions can we draw from this?

_____

_____

_____

Losing It for *Life*

Read again what Cathy wrote:

> Imagine living your life numb. Never really experiencing true happiness, joy, sadness, etc. In this state, life just sort of passes you by while you exist. Sadly enough, this is how I have lived most of my life. . . . This was the way I protected myself from past hurts, humiliations, letdowns, and unforgiveness in my life. The good news is that with the Lord's constant guiding in this journey, I have made a U-turn. Let me tell you, it is an incredible thing to feel, to really live life experiencing the good and the not-so-good times. It is so much better than simply existing in a numb state, day after day after day.

Do you relate to Cathy's experience? Are you numb much of the time? What sense does it make to let ourselves feel—fully embrace—painful feelings? What is the danger if we don't?

LOSE IT
for
LIFE

PART 2

_____

_____

_____

_____

Many overeaters are unaware that unidentified and unprocessed emotions are at the root of their hunger. Based on the twenty questions given in chapter seven, take the following self-test to see if you are an emotional eater.[1] Check all the boxes that apply.

❏ I think about food often or all the time.
❏ I eat to relieve tension, worry or upset feelings.
❏ I eat when I am bored.
❏ I continue to eat after I feel full, sometimes to the point of feeling sick.
❏ I use eating to relieve anxiety.
❏ I eat without thinking.
❏ I feel I have to clean my plate.
❏ I eat in secret or hide food.
❏ I eat quickly, shoveling in the food.
❏ I feel guilty after I eat.
❏ I eat small portions in front of people, but go back for more food when people aren't around.
❏ I binge (eat large amounts of food in a short period of time).
❏ I seldom eat one serving; instead I eat the entire amount (for example, a bag of cookies, a half-gallon of ice cream, and so forth).
❏ I feel out of control and impulsive when eating.
❏ I eat when I am not physically hungry.
❏ I lie to myself about how much I really eat.
❏ I have trouble tolerating negative feelings.
❏ I have impulse problems in other areas of my life (shopping, gambling, sex, alcohol, pornography, drugs, and so forth).
❏ I have been on numerous diets over the years.
❏ I experience constant weight fluctuations.

If you checked a number of those boxes, you are probably an emotional eater. This means that non-physical feelings often trigger your desire to eat. *When* you stop eating depends on *why* you are eating.

Is all this discussion of emotional eating a new thought to you? What do you think of the idea that food can be used as a comfort, a way of calming anxiety or numbing out trauma? How might a childhood

LOSE IT
for
LIFE

PART 2

Emotional pain can lead us down the road to anxiety, depression and eating problems if not handled well. It is our response to emotional pain that matters.

of physical or sexual abuse, growing up in the home of an alcoholic or mentally ill parent, push someone in this direction?

_____

_____

_____

The authors tell about Dr. Paul Brand, a man who dedicated his life to helping people with leprosy. His discovery? Leprosy is disfiguring because its victims are unable to feel pain. His conclusion? Pain is God's warning signal to us that something is wrong. His commitment? Dr. Brand spent his life trying to find a way to give his patients the "gift of pain."

Have you ever thought of pain as a "gift"? What sort of hidden blessings might be lurking within and behind emotional pain?

_____

_____

_____

Do you mostly control your emotions or do they mostly control you? Why?

_____

_____

_____

What would you say to the person who looks disapprovingly at "all that feelings stuff" and says, "We're supposed to forget what lies behind and press on to what lies ahead. It does no good to dredge up the past. Besides, you can't change things that have already taken place"?

_____

_____

_____

We've seen that God can be trusted to understand us and help us. How can other people also come alongside us and walk with us through emotionally hard times? Write about a time when friends did this for you.

_____

_____

_____

DAY 2:
Identifying Feelings (Part 1)

P A R T   2

In this chapter, we are focusing on eating as a response to negative feelings or emotional pain. Physical hunger is almost never the trigger for overeating. Overeating is typically a combustible combination of disturbing feelings and wrong thoughts, coupled with deeply ingrained behavior patterns and easily available food. What we must learn is: 1) How to identify the emotions associated with urges to overeat. 2) How to feel those emotions and manage them instead of allowing them to manage us. 3) How to work through emotional pain, grieve it, and allow God to transform it—and us.

Emotions aren't wrong or bad. What you do with an emotion is what counts. The work is to first acknowledge what emotion is triggering you.

Looking at Your *Life*

Jot down a few details and/or recollections about each of the following. When was the last time you . . .

cried?

_____

got really furious?

_____

felt really scared?

_____

were overcome by anxiety?

_____

felt genuinely depressed?

_____

sensed deep envy in your heart?

_____

were filled with guilt or shame?

_____

_____

What one emotion seems to keep popping up in your life more than others? What's your best guess as to what this is about?

_____

_____

LOSE IT *for* **LIFE**

PART 2

If you struggle with clinical depression, there is nothing wrong with taking an anti-depressant to help stabilize your mood and correct brain chemistry. You may need to see a doctor and/or therapist to help with depression.

Learning a New Way of *Life*

When you have the urge to eat, try to identify what you feel. This sounds simple but may not be if you were taught not to feel, or even to acknowledge negative emotions like anger, pride, envy and such. And yet, negative emotions are part of our human condition and must be dealt with in a healthy and biblical way.

Many people are surprised when they realize how often emotions are named and discussed in the Bible. Spend a few minutes reading and thinking your way through the following passages and questions.

What do you think of the statement that *anger* is the most reported emotion tied to overeating? How, if at all, have you seen this in your experience?

_____

_____

_____

The Bible says, "Be angry and do not sin" (Ephesians 4:26 NKJV). How is this possible?

_____

_____

The authors say that many of us overeat when we are *fatigued*. They suggest: "If you are tired, rest is what you need." Do you see this habit in your life? Read the following Scriptures that speak to the importance of rest. Then jot down the "big idea" of each passage.

Psalm 37:7

_____

_____

Matthew 11:28–30

_____

_____

Psalm 43 is only five verses long, but it gives insight into the single best way to overcome feelings of *depression*. Ponder the passage for a few minutes. Why is food an inadequate answer to feelings of depression?

_____

_____

When we are *lonely*, why are we inclined to seek out food instead of the people who could help address our loneliness? What does Psalm 68:6 say about this? How can a *spiritual* family help in these times?

_____

_____

If you sometimes eat because of feelings of *insecurity*, how do the words of Jesus in John 10:27–30 give you new hope and confidence?

_____

_____

Do you struggle with feelings of *guilt* and *shame*? Why? How does Romans 8:1–2 speak to your situation?

_____

_____

Losing It for *Life*

What new insights have you discovered into why you sometimes overeat?

_____

_____

Let's get practical and make a plan. The next time you feel strong anger or anxiety or some other uncomfortable feeling, what specific steps can you take to avoid turning to food to numb your pain?

_____

_____

TO DO: Show your plan to two trusted friends. Ask for their honest feedback. Pray *with* them and ask them to pray faithfully *for* you. Ask them to be your safety net of accountability.

Try this. Listen to some praise CDs in your car or home stereo system. Really pay attention to the lyrics. Test the adage that praise is the antidote to feeling down. Record your experience here.

_____

_____

Here's another valuable project: Make a list of your strengths and weaknesses. Thank God for the things you are able to do well. Then ask God to help you with your weaknesses. By His Spirit, He is able to accomplish much, even with our limitations (Zechariah 4:6).

Guilt is only healthy when it relates to sin. We should feel guilty when we disobey God's Word. But once we confess that sin, it is gone and forgotten.

Shame often develops from a message that you are bad, weak, or unloved. Yet Jesus does not shame you or judge you by your weight or your failures.

119

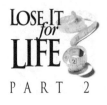

DAY 3:
Identifying Feelings (Part 2)

This set of workbook lessons explores the various ways in which we often eat to combat or to numb troubling feelings. We're learning that food isn't the answer. It might give us a brief bit of comfort or distraction, but it doesn't address the deepest needs of our hearts.

If you are willing to take your hurts and pains to Christ and lay them at His feet, . . . if you will refuse to believe the lies of the evil one, the food handcuffs will drop off you.

Looking at Your *Life*

As the LIFL book demonstrates, everyone has painful childhood memories—sad stories of betrayal or abandonment or abuse. The problem here is that when we suffer deep wounds as children, we simply don't have the vocabularies, life experience, opportunities, or tools to properly process these confusing events. Consequently they lodge in our souls and become defining. After such episodes of deep hurt or loss, we typically form wrong conclusions about God, others, and ourselves. Even worse, we vow to do whatever it takes to avoid feeling pain again. The result is a life of running and hiding, feeling numb, and doing everything we can to avoid trusting God or others.

Can you relate? Does this summary "ring true" in your own experience?

_____

_____

Take a big step of faith, and list your top five hurts or disappointments. What events have most deeply marked you? (Note: The goal here is not to wallow in misery, but to uncover clues to the mystery of who you are and why you function as you do.)

1. _____

2. _____

3. _____

4. _____

5. _____

Learning a New Way of *Life*

Before we look at some more emotional reasons people turn to food and end up overeating, consider this passage from the Gospel of Luke. It's interesting and relevant because it occurs right at the beginning of Christ's ministry. Notice how He describes His mission.

When the devil had finished all this tempting, he left [Jesus] until an opportune time. Jesus returned to Galilee in the power of the Spirit, and news about him spread through the whole countryside. He taught in their synagogues, and everyone praised him.

He went to Nazareth, where he had been brought up, and on the Sabbath day he went into the synagogue, as was his custom. And he stood up to read. The scroll of the prophet Isaiah was handed to him. Unrolling it, he found the place where it is written:

"The Spirit of the Lord is on me, because he has anointed me to preach good news to the poor. He has sent me to proclaim freedom for the prisoners and recovery of sight for the blind, to release the oppressed, to proclaim the year of the Lord's favor."

Then he rolled up the scroll, gave it back to the attendant and sat down. The eyes of everyone in the synagogue were fastened on him, and he began by saying to them, "Today this scripture is fulfilled in your hearing" (Luke 4:13–21).

LOSE IT *for* LIFE

P A R T   2

If you eat because you feel insecure, no amount of food will change that feeling. The only place you are truly secure is in your relationship with God.

What is significant about these phrases in the Isaiah passage that Jesus applied to himself?

- "freedom for the prisoners"

_____

_____

- "recovery of sight for the blind"

_____

_____

- "release the oppressed"

_____

_____

In what ways is food sometimes like a prison? How do we become oppressed by our eating habits and weight?

_____

_____

The LIFL book suggests that *jealousy* (comparing ourselves to others) can tempt us to eat when we're not really physically hungry. How so?

_____

_____

If you are one who eats when you are *happy*, what are some other ways you can celebrate (other than eating)?

_____

_____

LOSE IT for LIFE

PART 2

Eating is a great way to delay unpleasant tasks or waste time. But the task will still be there when you finish eating. It's best to tackle tough tasks head on.

Read the following passages that speak about *worry* or *fear*. What do you see in these verses that can help in your dieting?

Matthew 6:25–34

_____

_____

Philippians 4:6–7

_____

_____

What's the problem with being a nervous eater?

_____

_____

Losing It for *Life*

Spend a few minutes writing out responses to how emotions affect your eating habits. Then brainstorm some options.

Emotion	How This Prompts Me to Overeat	Some Options Instead of Food
Disappointment/Hurt		
Emptiness		
Procrastination		
Boredom		
Rejection		
Loss of control		

With which of the above emotions do you seem to struggle most?

_____

_____

Write candidly about a vivid personal experience of rejection.

_____

_____

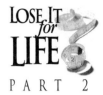

When people continually hurt you or let you down, food can easily become a trusted friend. It is always available. It tastes good and satisfies for the moment. But no matter how many times we turn to food, the pain won't go away. The hurt stays buried beneath increasing layers of fat. The authors write:

> To be healed, you must face rejection. Feel it with all your soul. Pour out your heart to the Lord. Once you've allowed yourself to really feel the pain of rejection, pray and ask God to take it. Then, ask Christ to speak His truth to you. You see, the enemy uses emotional pain to implant lies— no one will want or love you; people will only hurt you; if only you were thinner . . . all lies!
>
> The truth is that there is someone who will never reject you and is completely trustworthy. Your acceptance has nothing to do with your actions or your weight. Jesus unconditionally loves you because you are His. Know that Jesus Christ identifies with your pain. According to Isaiah 53, He was despised, rejected, and a man of sorrow. Because of His great love for you, He suffered the pain of rejection. On the cross, it was crucified once and for all. Once you allow His truth to soak your spirit, you can give up the pain of rejection and accept God's unfailing love.

Comment about how this passage speaks to you, how it effects you. Does their advice seem crazy?

_____

_____

Remembering the words of Christ in Luke 4 about freedom, write a prayer expressing your desire to be delivered from the grips of emotional eating.

_____

_____

Isn't it interesting that when we feel out of control, we eat out of control? You are not in control, so you might as well surrender to the One who is.

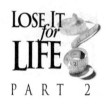

DAY 4:
Expressing Your Feelings

Once you've identified your feelings, you must learn to express them directly rather than medicating them with food.

So far we've seen that, like it or not, we are emotional creatures. All sorts of feelings permeate our souls. These feelings aren't inherently wrong, but if we're not careful, we can let them propel us in unhealthy directions. The fact is much overeating is due to the fact that we fail to understand, identify, and process disturbing emotions. We substitute food for feeling our feelings.

After looking at the most common culprits behind emotional eating, now we want to spend a session coming to grips with how to properly express our feelings. In times of strong emotion, the answer isn't to *take food in* but to *get our feelings out*!

Looking at Your *Life*

How hard is it for you to put words to what you're feeling? Did you grow up in a home where this expression was encouraged?

_____

_____

_____

Can you name your emotions? From the following list, circle the words that best describe how you feel right now. What's stirring in you?

Tired	Anxious	Alive
Irritated	Rejected	Joyful
Lonely	Vulnerable	Confused
Bored	Fragile	Stressed
Frustrated	Sad	Depressed
Guilty	Ugly	Discouraged
Scared	Compassionate	Encouraged
Jealous	Hopeful	Torn
Disconnected	Peaceful	
Worried	Hopeless	

Describe a life in which you were no longer at the mercy of powerful emotional urges. What might that be like? Why would that be preferable to your current lifestyle? How specifically would your daily experience be different?

_____

_____

_____

LOSE IT
for
LIFE

PART 2

Determine if there is a need behind what you're feeling; for example, the need to be loved, accepted, approved of, or respected.

Learning a New Way of *Life*

The Psalms are like a kind of textbook for learning how to process our feelings. Read Psalms 4–6. What do you observe? Does David seem like a guy who has difficulty admitting the struggles of his life and heart? Do you sense a hesitation in him to articulate the negative feelings he's experiencing? What's the implication for us?

_____

_____

_____

_____

See if you can list ten different ways feelings can be expressed. Which of these do you already do? Which would take some "getting used to"?

_____

_____

_____

Why do the authors place such emphasis on *confession;* that is, being honest about what is going on inside of you? (Hint: See Psalm 32:3.)

_____

_____

_____

_____

What are the dangers and pitfalls of not being upfront with others about our struggles, doubts, and failures? How does James 5:16 add to your understanding?

_____

_____

_____

LOSE IT for LIFE
PART 2

By breaking our silence and speaking the truth about ourselves aloud to God and another person, we move out of the darkness and bring secrets into the light.

If you want to break free from emotional eating, you must confess the need that is not being met and be honest about what you truly feel. Honesty brings about authentic change.

What ingredients create an atmosphere in which confession is more likely among Christian friends?

_____

_____

_____

_____

What character qualities should we look for in a confessor/confidante/accountability partner?

_____

_____

_____

_____

Losing It for *Life*

The authors say that *confession* means that we:

_____ submit ourselves to God's ways of handling secrets, respecting His desire for openness and vulnerability among His people.

_____ are willing to overcome our fear of rejection by revealing our failures to another person.

_____ reject our habit of self-protective secretiveness.

_____ admit to at least one other person that we have fallen short of God's best, including our character defects and judgment errors.

_____ have stopped trying to mask our true feelings.

_____ have chosen to humble ourselves before God and others.

_____ renounce our independence and admit that we need help from fellow believers.

_____ put our vague sense of guilt into written or spoken words and express the situation without making excuses.

Go back through this list and put a check mark before the actions you have done or are willing to do. Leave empty the blanks in front of the action steps that you still need to take.

Why do some of the steps seem harder to you than others?

_____

_____

_____

_____

_____

Begin to develop the skill of healthily expressing your feelings. A good pattern to follow (until you get comfortable) is to say and/or pray the following:

God, I feel _____ (name the emotion), *I think because* _____ (describe the situation or event that may have triggered the feeling). *But the truth about my situation is* _____ (remind yourself of pertinent facts and promises of God's Word). *O, Lord, renew my mind. Help me to see this situation through your eyes. Please give me the grace to cling to you. Grant me the courage to live by what you say is true, not by how I feel.*

Try saying this prayer right now.

Why is it wise to have more than one person to talk with about your struggles?

_____

_____

_____

_____

LOSE IT
for
LIFE

PART 2

God wants us to come to Him no matter what. Don't allow your losses and pain to turn you away from Him.

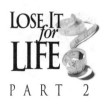

LOSE IT for LIFE
PART 2

When a highly stressful period hits, put a time limit on the amount of time you'll give to thinking about it.

DAY 5:
Reducing Stress

Stress can trigger overeating. If you remember from chapter 2, triggers (subtle or overt) always precede the urge to overeat. A trigger or cue can be a specific event or a person, or a feeling that arises from involvement in certain events or with certain people.

In this lesson we want to learn how to eliminate overeating triggers by reducing stress or avoiding certain events or people.

Looking at Your *Life*

During the last year, check which of the following stressful events you've experienced.

_____ death of a loved one	_____ death of a personal dream
_____ death of a friend	_____ termination of a friendship
_____ job loss	_____ financial setback
_____ change in jobs	_____ lifestyle change
_____ change in income	_____ surgery/hospitalization
_____ new home	_____ tax troubles
_____ new baby	_____ big vacation
_____ child moves out	_____ holiday with family
_____ change in marital status	_____ death of a pet
_____ new church	_____ automobile accident
_____ serious health issues	_____ home remodeling
_____ minor health issues	_____ natural disaster (flooding, fire, etc.)
_____ legal troubles	_____ other
_____ weight gain of more than 25 pounds	_____ NUMBER OF STRESSORS

1–3   Pray for the rest of us—that we don't become envious!
4–8   (sigh) Welcome to life in a fallen world.
9 or more   Bless your heart, "Job"!

Think about the people in your life. Which individuals leave you feeling stressed and tense—maybe because they engage you in certain conversations or bring up old memories? What precisely do they do?

_____

_____

What regular situations seem to get you agitated, so that you end up turning to food out of habit? Dissect those situations. What's really going on? What emotions do they stir within you?

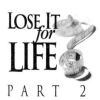

_____

_____

_____

Use this chart to list the stressful triggers that upset you and lead to overeating. Put them in the appropriate column. You can easily see which ones to eliminate, reduce or cope with in a different way.

Stress triggers to overeat	Can eliminate	Can reduce	Need new coping
EX: Lunch partners overeat	X		
Uncle Jim and politics		X	
Fights with spouse			X
Dealing with mother			X

Another great stress reducer is exercise. There is nothing like a relaxing game of golf, tennis, or racquetball to get your mind off the pressure through physical exertion.

Learning a New Way of *Life*

Read Psalm 13. What clues do you see here about David's situation? How does he go about handling his stress?

_____

_____

_____

Read Psalm 55. This is a lament of David in which he tells of betrayal at the hands of a close friend. What jumps out at you from this painful glimpse into David's "journal"? Was this an avoidable situation or one over which he had control?

_____

_____

What stresses in your life right now can't be eliminated? Instead of freaking out or bingeing on food, list some better options as you can for handling this stressful situation.

_____

_____

_____

LOSE It for LIFE
PART 2

Have you ever journaled? Do you now? If not, what do you think about this discipline? How could a prayer journal help you?

_____

_____

Losing It for _Life_

Assertiveness is simply standing up for what you know to be true and holding your position. In order to be assertive you have to know what you want and then verbalize it. You can't be afraid to hurt people's feelings. When you set a boundary or tell someone NO, they may get hurt, but that isn't your problem.

Are you the kind of person who feels pressured to please everyone, so that you take on more responsibility than you should? Give some examples. What responsibilities have you taken on that are now burdensome and stressful?

_____

_____

How can learning to say no become an effective tool in overcoming stress?

_____

_____

If you are someone who grew up in the home of an alcoholic, addicted, abusive, or mentally ill parent, chances are you really don't know how to relax. Why? Because growing up in a household in which peoples' moods and actions were unpredictable creates tension in children. Those tense kids become tense adults who never learned how to relax. Relaxation wasn't safe. Your guard had to be up or you could get hurt.

When—in the last five years—have you felt the most deeply relaxed?

_____

_____

What are some ways you'd love to learn to relax—if only you could give yourself permission to do so?

_____

_____

Pain is not optional, but misery is. You can't always control pain but you can do something about misery. If you are looking for a quick fix to emotional pain, find another book to read! We would rather you take this approach, "God's hand is upon me, and I am entering a process of healing—people to keep me accountable, support me, and confront me so I don't repeat the same mistakes along the way." Healing is often progressive because it requires changes in our character and actions. The way we cope with emotional pain must change if we decide to no longer eat our way through it.

Let's apply the RISE acronym to the issue of "emotional eating."

REDUCE: stress where and when you can; reduce eating in response to negative feelings and stress.

INCREASE: confession—your ability to stand and confront negative feelings and tough issues.

SUBSTITUTE: new ways—other than eating—to deal with painful emotions; feeling for running from feelings.

ELIMINATE: fear, stress whenever possible, feelings of rejection, and shame or hopelessness.

Keep a record of what you do when you become emotionally upset. You only have to record a few instances. Write down the event, the emotion and how you behaved or what you did. For example:

Event: Received an upsetting phone call from my ex.

Emotion: Very hurt.

Reaction: Went to the refrigerator and opened the door to eat.

Now, think of a new way to cope with that feeling. What could you substitute for eating? For example: *New behavior:* Call a friend and let her pray with me.

Here's another example:

Event: Heard someone gossip about me at church.

Emotion: Anger.

Reaction: Stopped at Wendy's for fries.

New behavior: Confronted the person who did the gossiping.

Make a list of ten behaviors you can substitute the next time you want to eat because of an intense emotion. Your list should include behaviors you can do while driving, at home, at work, and on the go. Post the list on your refrigerator and make a copy to take with you. Every time you are tempted to eat because you feel an unpleasant emotion, pull out your list and choose a new thing to do.

_____

_____

People who learn to respond to emotional pain without using food to numb themselves or to escape have a better and longer weight-loss maintenance record than those who only deal with eating and exercise. Both research and clinical experience support this idea. This work will be difficult because you'll be giving up a deeply ingrained way of coping. You may feel flooded with emotions that you haven't felt in a long time because eating has covered them up, but the rewards are well worth the effort. With God's help you can come out of the eating closet to a place of peace and rest.

Preparation: Read chapter eight of Lose It for Life *before you begin the lessons for Week 8.*

DAY 1:
Extreme Makeover

LOSE IT *for* LIFE

PART 2

What to Expect

Our culture is obsessed with "makeovers." Popular television shows document how people and houses undergo quick renovations. And, at least on the surface, the "before and after" differences *are* dramatic.

Our goal in this lesson is to focus on a deeper kind of makeover—one that starts in the heart and becomes a foundation for true, lasting change.

Looking at Your *Life*

List ten gadgets, products, trends, and so forth that suggest to you that people in our culture are only "skin deep" and obsessed with finding "the fountain of youth."

_____

_____

_____

So-called "reality shows" on television typically feature contestants who are physically attractive; yet, many of these people seem really shallow, self-absorbed, and vindictive. What does the emphasis on being outwardly attractive say to you?

_____

_____

Which of your physical features do you like best? Least? Why?

_____

_____

The world's foremost plastic surgeon calls you and says, "I'll perform any cosmetic procedure you desire, for free." How would you react? What kind of cosmetic alteration would you choose?

_____

_____

_____

Do you think television network executives would ever be interested in making a reality series about a group of Lose It For Life people deciding to lose weight? Why or why not? What features/underlying principles of LIFL might scare away the Hollywood crowd?

_____

_____

The truth is we all need an extreme makeover. The surgery required takes place in the heart. And the results last a lifetime.

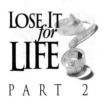

PART 2

Learning a New Way of *Life*

Speaking on behalf of those who know Jesus Christ by faith, the apostle Paul, wrote, "But we all, with unveiled face, beholding as in a mirror the glory of the Lord, are being transformed into the same image from glory to glory, just as by the Spirit of the Lord" (2 Corinthians 3:18).

What kind of transformation is this talking about? Put it into your own words.

_____

_____

_____

Read the following passages and jot down your thoughts after each one. Ask, "What does this say about God? About me? About how to change? What promise is here? What command?"

- "Those who become Christians become new persons. They are not the same anymore, for the old life is gone. A new life has begun!" (2 Corinthians 5:17 NLT)

_____

_____

- "Just as we are now like Adam, the man of the earth, so we will someday be like Christ, the man from heaven" (1 Corinthians 15:49 NLT).

_____

_____

- "Dear friends, now we are children of God, and what we will be has not yet been made known. But we know that when he appears, we shall be like him, for we shall see him as he is" (1 John 3:2).

_____

_____

What kind of makeover is God after? What kind of differences does he want to see in us?

_____

_____

How can deep change (insights, renovations at the soul level, and so forth) result in change at the surface level of *your* life (eating habits, weight, and others)?

_____

_____

_____

134

Losing It for *Life*

We need a deeper kind of makeover, the kind that originates in the soul and that lasts longer than a Botox injection or a facelift. One important step in the process is changing the way we think. Let's focus first on our *body image*.

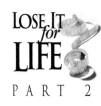

LOSE IT for LIFE

PART 2

Don't allow others to define you. Your identity must be fully secure in Christ.

Read Genesis 1:26–27 and Psalm 139. What is the message of these passages?

_____

_____

Whose image do you reflect? Should you try to meet society's warped, ever-morphing standards of beauty and fitness, or should you be content with the body you were given, making every effort to be in good health?

_____

_____

Can we ever get comfortable and okay—really and truly okay—with flawed bodies? How?

_____

_____

Think for a few moments about your *identity*. Write ten short phrases or one-word descriptions to answer the questions: "Who am I—really? What makes me significant?"

_____

_____

What would you say to the insecure teenager who is desperately relying on friends, looks, or talents to give him/her a sense of identity and significance? What's the flaw in this approach?

_____

_____

Now, let's focus on the subject of *personal worth*. We're not speaking here of net worth (as in money), but of worth in the sense of "where do I find value?" How would you answer the thoughtless person who insensitively says, "You're worthless—overweight, ugly and unloved. No one will *ever* care for you!"?

_____

_____

How do you know such a cruel remark is a total lie?

_____

_____

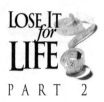

PART 2

*We will never
measure up
to the perfect
bodies plas-
tered on
billboards or
parading
around on TV.
It's time for all
of us to think
twice about
these messages
because they
impact our
lives in hugely
negative ways.*

Read through the following list of practices that can aid you in this lifelong process of "reprogramming your mind." How can these help you think and live in a way that honors God and brings joy? Write out your responses.

● Meditating on God's Word

_____

● Eating healthily

_____

● Exercising consistently

_____

● Doing realistic self-appraisals that involve more than just physical appearance

_____

● Focusing on becoming a person who is attractive internally

_____

● Learning to accept your body and what can't be changed

_____

● Refusing to compare ourselves with others; understanding that's God's plans and designs for each person are unique

_____

What is one big "take-away" truth you got from this lesson? How do you intend to put it into practice immediately?

_____

_____

_____

DAY 2:
Achieving Weightlessness

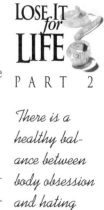

Negative body image is a modern-day plague tormenting many of us. But this doesn't have to be. One of the stated goals of Lose It For Life is to achieve a state of "weightlessness."

Looking at Your *Life*

How do you explain our culture's obsession with the human body? Why the relentless focus?

_____

_____

_____

What people do you know who really like their bodies and are content with the way they look?

_____

_____

_____

What about you? Write five words or phrases that describe how you honestly feel about your body.

_____

_____

_____

There is a healthy balance between body obsession and hating our bodies. Somewhere in the middle is acceptance and responsibility.

Learning a New Way of *Life*

In Lose It For Life lingo, "weightlessness" means you are *no longer defined by your weight.* How do you think someone gets to this place?

_____

_____

_____

The Bible says, "Don't you know that you yourselves are God's temple and that God's Spirit lives in you? If anyone destroys God's temple, God will destroy him; for God's temple is sacred, and you are that temple" (1 Corinthians 3:16–17). How can this truth alter the way we *view* our bodies? How can it affect the way we *treat* our bodies?

_____

_____

_____

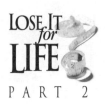

LOSE IT for LIFE

PART 2

Spend a few minutes pondering this ancient truth: "For as he thinks in his heart, so is he" (Proverbs 23:7 NKJV). What does this verse have to say to those who view their bodies with contempt?

_____

_____

_____

Think about the following people and situations:
- the overweight person who loudly and constantly jokes about how "fat" he or she is
- the young girl with the beautiful body who, because of emotional emptiness, gives herself sexually to every young man who comes along
- the individuals who make it their lifelong goal to look just like someone famous
- the people who spend hours daily pumping iron and admiring their mirrored, muscled images
- the heavy person who has a garage full of unused exercise equipment bought impulsively
- the hyper-kinetic young woman who exercises obsessively out of fear of gaining weight
- the anorexic model who is told she's a "cow" because her weight "ballooned" from 105 to 112 pounds

What common threads do you see in these behaviors?

_____

_____

_____

Which of these do you find the most understandable? The most bizarre? Why?

_____

_____

_____

Losing It for _Life_

Give yourself a much needed break! _Accept your body_, flaws and all, and care for it as the holy temple it is.

Why is it important to stop making degrading statements about how you look?

_____

_____

_____

The authors say: "Become your best encourager rather than your worst critic. That voice would say, 'You are overweight, but you're working on it.'"

Is being kind to yourself difficult for you? Why?

_____

_____

Some people put their life "on hold" until they are more comfortable with their body. What are the pitfalls of that kind of thinking?

_____

_____

Name three or four good positive qualities you have. Why is this sometimes hard to do?

_____

_____

In what ways can a person's weight or "oversized" body become a kind of mask?

_____

_____

The authors write: "Self-esteem is a misleading term. None of us can truly have esteem by looking to the *self*. The *self* is sinful, self-centered and easily deceived. God esteems you just because He chose and loves you. You don't have to earn His esteem. You already have it. Remember, He values you so much that He gave His only Son to die for you."

Do you agree with their assessment? Why or why not?

_____

_____

What truth or reminder in this lesson means the most to you and why?

_____

_____

LOSE IT for LIFE

PART 2

Our minds easily doubt God and can be deceived. Therefore we are to take each thought captive (2 Corinthians 10:5) and renew our minds with God's truth (Romans 12:2).

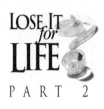

DAY 3:
Renewing the Mind

In this lesson, we want to look closely at the way we think. Consider this: Thoughts lead to feelings. Feelings lead to actions. Actions influence our perceptions that then influence our thoughts. It's a vicious cycle. What we think affects how we feel. And we eat in response to our feelings.

The bottom line? How and what we think—about life, God, ourselves, food—is crucial!

Looking at Your *Life*

Feelings are prompted by thoughts. For example, if you feel angry, it's because an angry thought preceded that feeling.

Give some examples from your own life from the last couple of days. Do a little soul-searching and record your thoughts below.

I found myself feeling . . .   **because (consciously or unconsciously) I was thinking . . .**
(EX: Depressed   *"I'll always be overweight and I'll never get married.")*

_____

_____

_____

Everyone engages in some kind of self-talk. That's where we say things to ourselves (or about ourselves), either out loud or internally. For example, a runner on the verge of exhaustion might say, "C'mon—keep going. You can do this!" A person who spills chili in his or her lap might blurt out through clenched teeth, "You idiot!"

Why do we do this "self-talk" thing? Where do you suppose we learned it? Why are some people so negative in what they say to themselves, while others are upbeat and positive?

_____

_____

_____

What about you? Describe your own self-talk habits. What kinds of remarks or statements do you find yourself speaking to yourself?

_____

_____

_____

Put yourself in each of the following situations and try to imagine what you would think, feel, and say.

LOSE IT
for
LIFE

PART 2

God knows and understands our thoughts. "You know my sitting down and rising up; You under- stand my thought afar off" (Psalm 139:2 NKJV).

If I . . .	I'd think . . .	I'd probably feel . . .	I'd likely say to myself . . .
Didn't get invited to an office party	EX: They don't like me because I'm fat	Embarrassed and angry	"When are you going to get off your butt and lose some weight?"
Heard someone make a "fat joke"			
Discovered I couldn't fit in a new outfit			
Strained a muscle try- ing to exercise			
Gave into the urge to eat a candy bar			
Were assigned to work with a good-looking, thin person			

Learning a New Way of *Life*

To paraphrase the noted author C. S. Lewis, people tend to make one of two mistakes in thinking about Satan, the evil one. Either they don't believe he is real, or they think they see demons behind every bush. Neither mindset is accurate. Jesus stated matter-of-factly: "The devil . . . was a murderer from the begin- ning, not holding to the truth, for there is no truth in him. When he lies, he speaks his native language, for he is a liar and the father of lies" (John 8:44).

How did Jesus view Satan? If the devil isn't real, what are we to conclude about Jesus?

_____

_____

_____

_____

141

LOSE IT
for
LIFE

PART 2

Whenever
something
negative or
traumatic
happens to us,
you can be
sure the enemy
uses that
situation to
implant a lie
and get us to
doubt God's
goodness.

Revelation 12:10 calls the devil "the accuser." 1 Peter 5:8 warns, "Be careful! Watch out for attacks from the Devil, your great enemy. He prowls around like a roaring lion, looking for some victim to devour" (NLT). From these descriptions, what conclusions can you draw about Satan? Is he benign?

_____

_____

_____

Read Ephesians 6:10–18. Notice that verse 16 says, "In every battle you will need faith as your shield to stop the fiery arrows aimed at you by Satan" (NLT). What do you think that phrase "fiery arrows" means? Is it possible that some of our persistent negative thoughts about ourselves might actually be whispered lies from the evil one?

_____

_____

_____

Losing It for *Life*

The New Testament book of Romans is often regarded as the most comprehensive, yet concise presentation of the Christian faith ever penned. Bible scholars note that the first eleven chapters of Paul's masterpiece are devoted to *what Christians should believe*, while the final five chapters focus on *how Christians should behave*.

Right at the hinge point between Paul's descriptions of right thinking and right living is this amazing verse: "Don't copy the behavior and customs of this world, but let God transform you into a new person by changing the way you think. Then you will know what God wants you to do, and you will know how good and pleasing and perfect his will really is" (Romans 12:2 NLT).

Older Bible translations refer to this process of changing the way we think as "renewing our minds." What does it mean to "renew" something?

_____

_____

_____

How do we renew our *minds*—begin to change the way we think, so that it ends up changing the way we live?

_____

_____

_____

Meditate for a few minutes on this verse:

> *"For My thoughts are not your thoughts,*
>
> *Nor are your ways, My ways, says the LORD.*
>
> *For as the heavens are higher than the earth,*
>
> *So are My ways higher than your ways,*
>
> *And My thoughts than your thoughts" (Isaiah 55:8–9 NKJV).*

The authors note that many times we become aware of a false way of thinking. We identify it (for example, "I realize I've been feeling all alone, . . . that no one cares for me") and perhaps we even know in our heads the truth of God ("Yet Jesus promised in Matthew 28 that he would never fail or leave his followers"). Still, sometimes, the truth isn't "real" to us. It doesn't seem at home in our hearts.

No amount of self-effort can make someone think differently. A renewed mind comes as we receive truth from God's Word.

What is the solution to this kind of disconnect? How do we get the truth of God to take root deeply in our souls?

_____

_____

_____

_____

The authors suggest the following practices and habits for beginning the lifelong process of "deprogramming and reprogramming" our minds. Think about each one and jot down why you think it is a valuable act.

- When you discover your heart is saying one thing and your head another, pray and ask Christ to speak His truth to you. Read His Word and ask Him to penetrate it deep into your mind and soul.

_____

_____

_____

- Skim the gospels. Notice that Jesus typically touched and healed broken bodies and souls (an experience) *while* also speaking truth to hurting and confused minds (cognitive). Why are both aspects important?

_____

_____

_____

_____

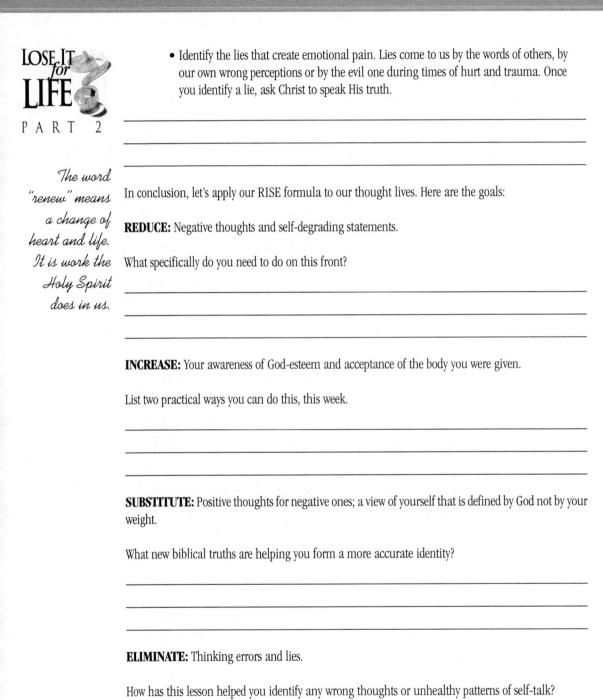

LOSE IT
for
LIFE
PART 2

The word "renew" means a change of heart and life. It is work the Holy Spirit does in us.

• Identify the lies that create emotional pain. Lies come to us by the words of others, by our own wrong perceptions or by the evil one during times of hurt and trauma. Once you identify a lie, ask Christ to speak His truth.

_____

_____

_____

In conclusion, let's apply our RISE formula to our thought lives. Here are the goals:

REDUCE: Negative thoughts and self-degrading statements.

What specifically do you need to do on this front?

_____

_____

_____

INCREASE: Your awareness of God-esteem and acceptance of the body you were given.

List two practical ways you can do this, this week.

_____

_____

_____

SUBSTITUTE: Positive thoughts for negative ones; a view of yourself that is defined by God not by your weight.

What new biblical truths are helping you form a more accurate identity?

_____

_____

_____

ELIMINATE: Thinking errors and lies.

How has this lesson helped you identify any wrong thoughts or unhealthy patterns of self-talk?

_____

_____

DAY 4:
Taking Negative Thoughts Captive

In order to lose it for life, you have to learn to identify negative and extreme thoughts, stop them from running rampant in your mind, and replace them with thoughts that are true and reflect who you are in Christ. That is the focus of this workbook lesson.

Looking at Your *Life*

When you were growing up, were your parents more optimistic or pessimistic?

_____

_____

_____

If your parents were critical or harsh, how did this contribute to your self-view?

_____

_____

_____

Describe your thought processes and mental habits by checking all that apply:

_____ I'm definitely scatterbrained.

_____ I have a mind like a steel trap; I remember most everything.

_____ My mind is always racing, juggling a zillion different things.

_____ No matter how crazy life gets, I am able to turn my brain off and just relax.

_____ I have a disciplined mind.

_____ I often have a different perspective on things, a different way of solving problems.

_____ I'm an outside-the-box thinker.

_____ Friends joke that I'm spacey or an airhead.

_____ People tell me I think too deeply, too much.

_____ The truth is I try not to think too much.

_____ It's hard for me to organize and articulate my thoughts.

_____ I daydream and fantasize a lot.

How do you typically respond when people ask, "What's on your mind?" or "A penny for your thoughts?"

_____

_____

_____

LOSE IT
for
LIFE
PART 2

"Since, then, you have been raised with Christ, set your hearts on things above, where Christ is seated at the right hand of God. Set your minds on things above, not on earthly things" (Colossians 3:1–2).

How much do you engage in "self-talk"? When life gets challenging or stressful what kinds of thoughts run through your mind? Are they mostly supportive and positive, or discouraging and negative?

_____

_____

_____

When you're not at work or on duty at home, where does your mind go? What kinds of daydreams do you have? Why?

_____

_____

_____

Why does it matter what we think?

_____

_____

Learning a New Way of *Life*

Second Corinthians 10:4–5 tells us to take our thoughts captive: "The weapons we fight with are not the weapons of the world. On the contrary, they have divine power to demolish strongholds. We demolish arguments and every pretension that sets itself up against the knowledge of God, and we take captive every thought to make it obedient to Christ."

The Message paraphrase puts it this way: "We use our powerful God-tools for smashing warped philosophies, tearing down barriers erected against the truth of God, fitting every loose thought and emotion and impulse into the structure of life shaped by Christ."

What does it mean to "take thoughts captive"? Why is this important?

_____

_____

_____

Picture your mind as the vital control center of your whole life. Now, picture inside your mind a shadowy and strong group of untrue, destructive thoughts and attitudes and conclusions—sort of mental terrorists. These bogus ways of thinking are loose inside your mind. Their goal? To wreak havoc. They want to get you to act in wrong ways by getting you to believe wrong ideas about God, the world, yourself, others, and so forth. Our only hope is to be alert and to begin the deliberate task of identifying, arresting, and replacing every one of these dangerous thoughts. If we don't, a full and rich life will elude us. If we don't, tragedy awaits.

Read Philippians 4:8. Why is this command so crucial?

_____

_____

_____

LOSE IT
for
LIFE

Give some examples of some common wrong, negative or degrading statements you find yourself saying to or about yourself. Then write out some positive, encouraging statements that need to be substituted.

A Thought that Needs to Be Replaced	**The Truth that Needs to Be Embraced**
1. EX: "I just ate all those cookies. I am so bad."	"I am not bad because Christ is in me. I am tempted and sometimes sin but when I do, I ask forgiveness and move on. I wish I hadn't eaten all those cookies but it's not the end of the world. I can regain control with God's help. Lord, give me the self-control I need right now."

Once we realize a thought is negative, self-degrading or untrue, we must move to stop the thought. To stop a thought, pretend you are grabbing it out of the air and taking it captive.

2. _____   2. _____

3. _____   3. _____

4. _____   4. _____

5. _____   5. _____

Losing It for *Life*

The authors say: "Sometimes it helps to put a rubber band on your wrist and snap it every time you tell yourself a negative thought or a lie. The mild pain is a simple reminder to grab the thought."

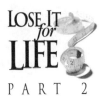

Do you think this would be an effective tool for change for you? Why or why not?

_____

_____

_____

What of the following is more common in your mind, and why?

- negative thoughts (pessimism)
- false beliefs (thoughts contrary to what God says is true)
- self-degrading sentences (condemning attacks on your own character or actions)

_____

_____

_____

In Appendix F of the *Lose It for Life* book, the authors recommend that you keep a Dysfunctional Thought Record (a chart designed to help people get in touch with their conscious and not-so-conscious thoughts). Simply record the date, briefly describe the situation, record what emotion you felt, and rate its intensity from 0–100 percent in terms of how intense that emotion felt. Next, record the automatic thought that came into your mind. Once you identify the thought and write it down, then try to think of a true thought and write that thought down. Then re-rate your emotion—it should be less intense. It might look like this:

Date	Situation	Emotion	Automatic Thought	Rational Response	Outcome
3/20	I over-ate	Disgust (80%)	*I am a loser*	"I blew it but can get back on track."	(10%)

EX: The situation was overeating. The emotion you record was *disgust* and you gave it an 80 percent rating, which means you felt it intensely. Your automatic thought was, *I am a loser.* The more rational response or truth is, "I blew it but can get back on track. It was only 10 cookies. I *am* weak in my own power, but with Christ I can do all things." Letting that truth sink in brings peace, so you re-rate your emotion to 10 percent.

Keeping such a chart will help you begin to recognize the thoughts that trigger your emotions. And you can review your thoughts and write alternative ways to think about situations.

What about *anxious* thinking. What is it? Is this a recurring problem for you? How does negative self-talk make things worse?

_____

_____

_____

List a couple of events, meetings, appointments or situations coming up in the next few days that make you feel anxious. Spend a few minutes trying to uncover the thoughts (or negative self-talk) behind your nervous feeling. Now, go back and put a more positive, more truthful spin on things.

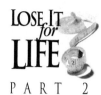

PART 2

Anxious thinking makes anxious people. Learn to take those thoughts captive and turn your thinking around.

_____

_____

_____

Review the following anxiety-thought checklist, and see if you think like an anxious person.

ANXIOUS-THOUGHT CHECKLIST

- ❑ I immediately think in terms of the "worst-case scenario."
- ❑ I am convinced I'm the next victim of every tragedy or illness.
- ❑ I focus on an unlikely problem, ignoring all the opposing data that suggests success.
- ❑ I interpret things in their worst possible light.
- ❑ I automatically believe nothing will change and I can't meet the challenge, so I just give up.
- ❑ I assume because something happened once, it will happen again.
- ❑ I believe things happen all the time or not at all.
- ❑ I am the classic perfectionist who doesn't allow for mistakes or human fallibility.
- ❑ I am extremely critical of myself and need to give myself a break!
- ❑ I am the classic "what if" worrier, who sees only possibilities for disaster or problems.

If you checked even a few of these statements, it's past time to change your thoughts. Think of the biggest challenge you are facing over the next month. First, write down your honest thoughts (even if they're negative) about that situation. Next, write down some positive, Scripture-based statements (like Philippians 4:13) to counter your anxious, negative thinking.

_____

_____

_____

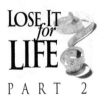

PART 2

DAY 5:
A New Attitude

In the last four lessons, we explored a number of life-changing truths. We've also proposed some exercises that—if practiced faithfully over time—can lead to a new way of thinking and living. In this lesson we want to tie up loose ends and make "renewing our mind" a regular, ongoing part of our lives.

Looking at Your *Life*

Sometimes life comes crashing down, and changes that we didn't want or expect are forced on us. Other times we choose to make changes. Which kind of change is harder? Give some examples of each from your own life.

_____

_____

_____

_____

Name a few helpful practices that are a part of your daily routine (for example, flossing my teeth). How and why did you develop this habit? How long did it take for you to make this a regular activity? How do you maintain the discipline to keep at it?

_____

_____

_____

_____

Why does the word *discipline* or the phrase "disciplining ourselves" have a nasty connotation to most people?

_____

_____

_____

As we've been examining the ways we think and the kinds of ideas and beliefs that drive us, what surprises you most? What have you learned about yourself?

_____

_____

_____

_____

"Worry is unproductive. I can't predict how life will go today and that is OK. I can live with uncertainty and change. God promises He won't give me anything I can't handle." (One lifelong worrier's new morning self-talk routine)

Learning a New Way of *Life*

In chapter eight of the LIFL book, we meet Rita, a woman controlled by worry. Find her brief story and review it. What about her experience speaks to you most powerfully?

_____

_____

_____

Read Matthew 4:1–11, the classic account of Christ's temptation. Theologically, this is a *profound* passage with infinite implications that make our finite brains dizzy. Practically, it can be argued this is a simple battle over what's true. In what ways do we fight the same sort of battle and face the same sort of choices every day?

_____

_____

_____

What can we learn here about the evil one?

_____

_____

_____

What can we learn *from* Christ in watching how he handles the tempter?

_____

_____

_____

In many of the apostle Paul's New Testament letters, he goes to great lengths laying out what Christians should *believe,* before telling them what they should do. Why do you think?

_____

_____

_____

Spend a few minutes pondering these passages that speak about the importance and the power of God's Word:

> *"How can a young man keep his way pure? By living according to your word. . . . I have hidden your word in my heart that I might not sin against you" (Psalm 119:9, 11).*

LOSE IT
for
LIFE

PART 2

"I have chosen the way of truth; I have set my heart on your laws" (Psalm 119:30).

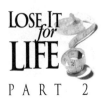

PART 2

"Your word is a lamp to my feet and a light for my path" (Psalm 119:105).

"All Scripture is God-breathed and is useful for teaching, rebuking, correcting and training in righteousness, so that the man of God may be thoroughly equipped for every good work" (2 Timothy 3:16–17).

According to these verses, what benefits do we get from knowing and following God's Word?

_____

_____

_____

Meditation is focusing your mind on things that bring peace and a sense of well-being. Think about God's intense love for you. Our God has promised to take care of us and meet all our needs. If that doesn't lessen your stress, nothing will.

Is it possible to live a healthy, productive, and fulfilling life apart from a deep knowledge of the truth of God? Why or why not?

_____

_____

_____

Losing It for *Life*

Noting that much stress originates from our own thought lives, the LIFL authors propose two strategies to help with stressful thoughts: (1) visualizing peaceful scenes and (2) meditating.

What is your immediate reaction to these suggestions?

_____

_____

_____

What does Philippians 4:8 suggest about meditation?

_____

_____

_____

_____

What is the promise of Isaiah 26:3? What guarantees peace?

_____

_____

_____

The authors write:

When you feel stressed and tense, you can also visualize yourself in a quiet peaceful place. This is calming. Some people like to imagine themselves resting on a sunny beach with a gentle breeze, the smell of the ocean, clear skies, and water. Other people find a mountain cabin in the snow to be a quiet, calming place. Others imagine basking eternally in the presence of Christ. I (Dr. Linda) like to read Revelation 21 and picture the New Jerusalem based on the visual description John gives in that chapter—the gates, the angels, the gems, but mostly the glory of God that will shine and illuminate the city! It doesn't matter what scene you choose, just think of something peaceful and try to engage all your senses in the scene. If you succeed, your anxious thoughts will melt as you settle into a place of peace.

How might this practice change your mindset and outlook in everyday life?

_____

_____

_____

Since God is the source of ultimate peace and serenity, how can thinking about Him (His goodness, His love, what He has done for you, the hope of His eternal presence, and so forth), bring about deep changes in our overall state of mind?

_____

_____

_____

As you engage in the Lose It For Life process, be prepared! You *will* hit bumps along the way related to how you think. It is easy to question God in times of difficulty, and it is easy to grow impatient and allow the enemy to gain ground in our thoughts. But God wants to teach us to depend on Him all the time, to renew our minds with His truth, and know that He is powerful and able to accomplish much in us if we submit to His plan.

Write out a short prayer to God summarizing all you are learning, thinking, feeling, and hoping. Ask Him to give you victory in the battle to renew your mind.

_____

_____

_____

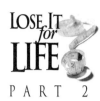

PART 2

We serve a God who raises the dead. Certainly He can resurrect our lives from defeat to new life with meaning and purpose.

Preparation: Read chapter nine of Lose It for Life *before you begin the lessons for Week 9.*

DAY 1:
Acting in the Truth

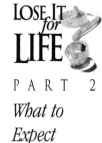

LOSE.IT
for
LIFE

PART 2

*What to
Expect*

Throughout the Lose It For Life program, we've been encouraging lifestyle changes. In this set of workbook lessons, we want to reinforce the need to make changes not only in the way you think and feel but also in the way you *behave.*

Looking at Your *Life*

How many diet or exercise books have you bought in your lifetime? How many have you actually read and tried to follow? How many are on your shelves or by your bedside?

_____

_____

*Good intentions
don't bring
success. Action
is required.*

A few years ago, an athletic shoe company saw sales skyrocket with an ad campaign built around the catch phrase "Just Do It." In what ways is this simple philosophy good and helpful? In what ways is it not helpful?

_____

_____

What are some right behaviors you have no problem doing?

_____

_____

What are some good and wise actions or habits you have to force yourself to do? Why?

_____

_____

For most people who battle with their weight, is the problem a lack of *information* or a lack of *application*? What about for you? Explain.

_____

_____

Learning a New Way of *Life*

Read this Scripture passage from the apostle Paul that discusses the difficulty of knowing the truth and acting in the truth:

*"What I don't understand about myself is that I decide one way, but then I act another,
doing things I absolutely despise. So if I can't be trusted to figure out what is best for*

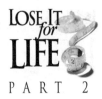

myself and then do it, it becomes obvious that God's command is necessary. But I need something more! For if I know the law but still can't keep it, and if the power of sin within me keeps sabotaging my best intentions, I obviously need help! I realize that I don't have what it takes. I can will it, but I can't do it. I decide to do good, but I don't really do it; I decide not to do bad, but then I do it anyway. My decisions, such as they are, don't result in actions. Something has gone wrong deep within me and gets the better of me every time" (Romans 7:15–20 THE MESSAGE).

Do you relate to Paul's honest admission? Pick a recurring temptation in your life, and record a bit of your own recent struggle.

_____

_____

How does a person move beyond good intentions to disciplined action and, ultimately, success?

_____

_____

What's the difference between trying really hard (good intentions, human willpower) and trusting God (faith)?

_____

_____

Knowing what we know about eating, exercising, and losing weight, we often try to will ourselves to do right and stay on our plan. Too often, we find ourselves doing what Paul says—the very things we say we won't do. We need something more.

Read Romans 10:17. What does it offer to this study?

_____

_____

Discuss your own current "intake" of the message of the Word of God.

_____

_____

Speaking of the need for action rooted in faith, the apostle James warned:

"Don't fool yourself into thinking that you are a listener when you are anything but, letting the Word go in one ear and out the other. Act on what you hear! Those who hear and don't act are like those who glance in the mirror, walk away, and two minutes later

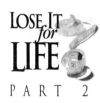

have no idea who they are, what they look like. But whoever catches a glimpse of the revealed counsel of God—the free life!—even out of the corner of his eye, and sticks with it, is no distracted scatterbrain but a man or woman of action. That person will find delight and affirmation in the action" (James 1:22–25 *The Message*).

What action is called for here?

_____

_____

What is promised to the person who takes decisive action?

_____

_____

God has already given you what you need to overcome. With the Holy Spirit operating in your life, you are empowered to do those things you know to be true.

Losing It for *Life*

As we saw above, we build a stronger faith in God by getting into His Word—or more precisely, by letting His Word get into us. Some ways God's truth can take root and bear fruit in our lives:

- hearing the Word preached (listening and taking notes)
- reading the Bible
- participating in small group Bible study
- studying the Bible for ourselves
- memorizing Bible passages
- meditating on Scripture (mulling it over in our minds; reflecting upon it's meaning and implications)

In which of these activities do you engage regularly?

_____

_____

_____

Which ones do you not do? Why?

_____

_____

Which ones do you want to learn how to do?

_____

_____

_____

LOSE IT for LIFE

PART 2

Even if you've had a history of weight loss failure, it's time to look forward and begin applying action to what you've read.

Answer the following questions by writing "Yes" or "No."

_____ Do you have a Lose It For Life support team?

_____ Do you have daily contact with your support team?

_____ Do you rely on your support team—calling them in times of weakness, etc.?

_____ Are you gut-level honest with your support team about your deep struggles and even your failures?

_____ Have you given your support team permission to ask you hard questions and tell you hard truths?

_____ Do you listen to your support team?

_____ When all is said and done, are you submitted to your support team (that is, would you follow their collective advice even if you didn't feel like it or want to)?

The more "no" answers you wrote, the less your chances of success. (See Proverbs 27:17.)

What's the truth or reminder you are taking away from this lesson?

_____

_____

Write a prayer expressing your need for God to work in you to "will and to act according to his good purpose" (Philippians 2:13).

_____

_____

DAY 2:
Tools for Change

Change is a process that involves multiple steps. In this lesson we will look at some helpful tools that—if used properly and consistently—can make your goal of losing it for life a reality.

Looking at Your *Life*

Thinking back over the last five years, what technology, insight, or learned skill has resulted in the greatest positive change in your life?

_____

_____

What's the most helpful tool you own and use regularly? Why is it such a favorite of yours?

_____

_____

_____

What tool or gadget or gizmo do you *not* have that you feel certain would make your life better, easier, or richer? Why?

_____

_____

_____

Play counselor for a moment to people desirous of change. A smoker friend asks, "How can I stop?" What counsel would you give?

_____

_____

_____

A family member in financial distress sighs, "We need a miracle . . . " What advice would you offer?

_____

_____

A colleague at work laments the moral condition of our nation and wonders aloud, "Will things ever change?" What do you say in response?

_____

_____

_____

LOSE IT
for
LIFE

PART 2

Overwhelmed? Don't worry. No one expects you to make all the changes at once.

PART 2

Motivation comes when you understand that the life God has for you is beyond what you could even imagine. God doesn't want you immobilized by your weight.

Learning a New Way of *Life*

Chapter nine of *Lose It for Life* suggests six steps that can be tools for change. Based on the discussion of these concepts from the book, write a brief definition or description of each.

Illumination— _____

Inspiration— _____

Examination— _____

Motivation— _____

Determination— _____

Realization— _____

Ephesians 5:8 says,

> "You groped your way through that murk once, but no longer. You're out in the open now. The bright light of Christ makes your way plain. So no more stumbling around. Get on with it!" (*THE MESSAGE*)

What does this verse tell us about the concept of *illumination*?

_____

_____

_____

The apostle Paul warned:

> "Don't become so well-adjusted to your culture that you fit into it without even thinking. Instead, fix your attention on God. You'll be changed from the inside out. Readily recognize what he wants from you, and quickly respond to it. Unlike the culture around you, always dragging you down to its level of immaturity, God brings the best out of you, develops well-formed maturity in you" (Romans 12:2 *THE MESSAGE*).

What do this verse suggest about the source of *inspiration*?

_____

_____

Read Psalm 139:23–24. What do these verses say about the process of *examination*?

_____

_____

_____

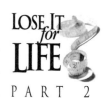

In what ways is taking a hard look at one's true condition terrifying? Why is this scary step so crucial?

_____

_____

_____

How can comparing ourselves with others be demotivating?

_____

_____

If you fall down and blow it, get up and try again. God gives us second chances. He wants us to succeed.

Losing It for *Life*

If illumination means seeing the need for change, describe the *illumination* that has taken place in your life so far in the LIFL program?

_____

_____

What is your current *inspiration* level? How would you say God has worked and is working within you to prompt long-term lifestyle changes?

_____

_____

Socrates said, "An unexamined life is not worth living." How and when do you regularly assess yourself—your heart, your motives, your attitudes, and your actions?

_____

_____

Other than God's Word, what other sources of feedback help you know where you are and how you're progressing?

_____

_____

Colossians 3:12 tells us how to dress for success: "So, chosen by God for this new life of love, dress in the wardrobe God picked out for you: compassion, kindness, humility, quiet strength, discipline" (THE MESSAGE).

How does a person do this? What role does the Spirit of God play in this process?

_____

_____

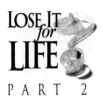

How can these internal qualities or tools make a difference in your external appearance?

_____

_____

_____

Luke 18 tells about Jesus encountering a desperate blind man and asking him an amazing question: "What do you want me to do for you?" Imagine yourself at Jesus' feet and hearing Him ask you the same thing. Dream big. Don't be superficial and ask just for a thin physique. What do you want—really want—in your deep heart? How would you like Him to transform who you are?

_____

_____

_____

Illumination, inspiration, examination, motivation, determination, and realization. Take some time to pray these tools of change into your life. Talk to God about each one.

DAY 3:
You Can Do It!

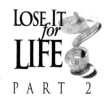

The goal of this short lesson is to bolster our faith and our resolve by remembering the limitless power and grace and goodness of our God.

With Christ, all things are possible. Stay in the fight and keep reaching for the prize.

Looking at Your *Life*

What is your greatest accomplishment in life—your proudest achievement? How did you do it?

_____

_____

What lessons did this experience teach you?

_____

_____

What positive, upbeat people do you admire and like to be around?

_____

_____

_____

How did they develop such an up, can-do attitude?

_____

_____

_____

What's the difference between "faith that can move mountains" and everyday "positive thinking" that doesn't necessarily involve God?

_____

_____

_____

It's been said, "If you have a little God, you'll have big problems. But if you have a big God, you'll have little problems." Why is one's view of God so important in life?

_____

_____

_____

LOSE IT
for
LIFE

PART 2

Learning a New Way of *Life*

James 1:12 says, "Anyone who meets a testing challenge head-on and manages to stick it out is mighty fortunate. For such persons loyally in love with God, the reward is life and more life" (THE MESSAGE). What rewards await the person who drops 50 pounds?

_____

_____

What rewards await the person who drops 50 pounds *and* who also undergoes radical changes in the way he or she thinks about God, self, food, and exercise?

_____

_____

_____

Ephesians 3:20 remind us, "God can do anything, you know—far more than you could ever imagine or guess or request in your wildest dreams! He does it not by pushing us around but by working within us, his Spirit deeply and gently within us" (THE MESSAGE).

Spend a few minutes meditating upon these Bible passages:

> *"Is anything too hard for the LORD?" (Genesis 18:14).*

> *"Ah, Sovereign LORD, you have made the heavens and the earth by your great power and outstretched arm. Nothing is too hard for you" (Jeremiah 32:17).*

> *"I am the LORD, the God of all mankind. Is anything too hard for me?" (Jeremiah 32:27).*

> *"I tell you the truth, if you have faith as small as a mustard seed, you can say to this mountain, 'Move from here to there' and it will move. Nothing will be impossible for you" (Matthew 17:20).*

> *Jesus replied, "What is impossible with men is possible with God" (Luke 18:27).*

Jot down your observations and insights from these verses.

_____

_____

A wise old saint once said, "Expect great things from God; attempt great things for God." What great things would you love to see God do *in* you?

_____

_____

_____

What "impossible" things would you love to see God do *through* you?

_____

_____

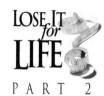

Losing It for *Life*

When Jesus began his public ministry at age 30, he went to the synagogue in his hometown of Nazareth (see Luke 4:16–21). He read a passage from Isaiah 61:1–2, in essence saying that his ministry would involve these activities.

*"The Spirit of the Sovereign L*ORD *is on me,*
*because the L*ORD *has anointed me to preach good news to the poor.*
He has sent me to bind up the brokenhearted,
to proclaim freedom for the captives
and release from darkness for the prisoners,
*to proclaim the year of the L*ORD'*s favor."*

Supernatural things can happen. Persevere until change comes.

Look at the phrases that Jesus quoted. What do you need him to do in your life?

_____

_____

The issue really isn't how much faith we have; it's who or what we have our faith in. How has your trust in God's character and power grown during your LIFL experience?

_____

_____

Assorted voices (internal and external) call out to us each day—mocking us, discouraging us, and trying to dampen our faith. What negative voices ring out loudest in your ears?

_____

_____

What can you do to stand strong on the truth of God's Word in a noisy world filled with lies?

_____

_____

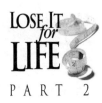

DAY 4:
Food in Social Settings?

Previously we talked about eating in response to specific *emotions* such as anger, boredom, guilt, and others, as well as eating triggered by specific negative *thoughts* (for example, "I am a loser," "I might as well eat because nothing I do ever succeeds anyway," "This is too difficult," and so forth). In this lesson, we want to examine another cue that triggers overeating: the social cue.

Looking at Your *Life*

When you're on a trip or vacation, what restaurants do you stop at most and why?

_____

_____

How susceptible are you to food advertisements on television? When did a billboard or commercial prompt you to head straight for a restaurant?

_____

_____

Do you tend to eat more when you are alone, or when you're in a public setting where there is a lot of food? Why?

_____

_____

Rank the following social food settings/scenarios from 1–10, with 1 = "the least tempting" and 10 = "an almost certain overeating disaster."

_____ You go in the break room at work, and a grateful client or supplier has sent over a giant cookie basket.

_____ At a small group social, the host's dining room table is overflowing with rich, fatty finger foods.

_____ The church has a big potluck dinner and each woman has rolled out a heaping helping of her best recipe.

_____ It's late night—you're restless, and a commercial for your favorite fast food restaurant (which is only half a mile from your house) comes on TV.

_____ The whole family is sitting down to a sumptuous Thanksgiving feast with all your holiday favorites.

_____ Your co-workers ask you to lunch, and they choose your favorite pizza buffet.

_____ You realize you need to run to the grocery store—and you are also *starving*!

_____ At a kid's birthday party in a popular fast food restaurant, you notice your child's "kiddie meal" has been all but ignored, leaving you staring at a tray full of tempting fries, cheeseburger, and chocolate shake to boot!

_____ A lavish wedding reception features several tables of exotic seafood dishes you don't normally get to sample.

_____ Visiting friends insist that you keep all the leftover yummies from a spontaneous cook-out/pitch-in dinner.

Learning a New Way of *Life*

Social cues are triggers in your living or working environment that increase your likelihood of overeating.

Upon rebuilding the walls of Jerusalem, Governor Nehemiah had Ezra the scribe come and read the Law of God, while the Levites explained it's meaning to the Jewish people. Upon hearing God's Word, the people were convicted about their sin and failure to live as they should. They were weeping as they listened. But then Nehemiah said, "Go and enjoy choice food and sweet drinks, and send some to those who have nothing prepared. This day is sacred to our Lord. Do not grieve, for the joy of the LORD is your strength" (Nehemiah 8:10).

What does this event suggest about eating and celebrating together with others?

_____

_____

The authors say: "The best way to handle commercials, especially late night when you are tired and your defenses are down, is to use the remote to click past the commercials. Don't watch them and you won't be triggered. And certainly don't watch food channels or cooking shows. Both can trigger a desire to overeat."

Has this food commercial trigger been a problem for you? How so?

_____

_____

Proverbs 19:20 says: "Listen to advice and accept instruction, and in the end you will be wise." Read the following tidbits of advice and instruction from chapter nine of *Lose It for Life*. Then jot down your initial honest responses to each.

1. "This association of the car with eating must be broken. The best way to do this is not to eat in the car at all. We know that sounds impossible to some of you. . . . Relegate all eating to the kitchen table."

_____

_____

2. "Movies can be very enjoyable without the snacks. Drink a full glass of water before you go or eat a low cal snack so the sight and smell of all those goodies won't be so tempting. You've learned to associate eating with movies. Now you have to unlearn that behavior."

_____

_____

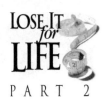

3. "If you are asked to bring food to an event, bring something healthy you can snack on, and park your body close to that snack food. . . . You can hold a glass of punch or diet drink in one hand for a long time while you are busy making conversation and interacting with new people."

_____

_____

4. "Look around your workplace. Are there places in that setting that trigger eating? How about the coffee pot? It can be a place of gathering and snacking. . . . You may have to skip the coffee pot and socialize by the water fountain instead."

_____

_____

5. "Eat before you grocery shop. This also helps cut down on buying impulse items. . . . Avoid the cookie aisle and prepackaged foods that are high in trans fat."

_____

_____

6. "You must break the habit of tasting and eating while cooking. . . . Ask someone else to taste the stew if you think it may need more salt. Stir the pot and put down the spoon. . . . And during cleanup, don't eat the extras on peoples' plates. You have to be comfortable throwing food away."

_____

_____

7. "Use foil wrap for leftover foods. When you don't see what the dish is, it isn't as tempting to eat it."

_____

_____

Proverbs 21:5 says: "The plans of the diligent lead to profit as surely as haste leads to poverty." How, specifically and practically, can advance planning help you avoid overeating in social situations?

_____

_____

_____

What would it be like and how might it work if you planned the next day's "menu" (or approved eating list) each night before you went to bed?

_____

_____

Losing It for *Life*

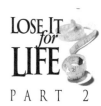

LOSE IT
for
LIFE
PART 2

No one can make all these changes at once. It's a good idea to begin with something small. What one thing will you choose to do differently for a month? Write that commitment down, and begin by making that change.

_____

_____

Try to think which social situations or cues trigger you to overeat. Then problem solve ahead of time how you will handle that situation.

Research experts tell us that it takes three weeks to a month to learn a new habit and make it a part of our routine. Theoretically, then, someone serious about making lifestyle eating and exercise changes could develop *twelve new habits a year*.

What twelve small changes would you like to see in your life? Be specific. Write them down.

_____

_____

Now, look into the future and imagine how these new lifestyle patterns could add up to make your life experience richer. Record your hopes and dreams here.

_____

_____

Remember, make one small behavior change your goal for each month. Keep adding changes as you are able. If you fail, cut yourself a break. Keep plodding. Eventually these small changes will add up. If you took years to put on the weight, give yourself time to take it off.

Usually if you take something away, you need to replace it with something else. Otherwise most of us will merely substitute another problem-behavior in its place. (For example, maybe you have stopped overeating but now notice you're beginning to overspend.)

When has this kind of problem substitution been the case with you?

_____

_____

Your goal is to eat for nourishment and the enjoyment of meals. It is up to you to discover the other illegitimate function that eating has served in your life. Some of those wrong functions are using food to calm yourself, to relax, to numb you, to boost your mood, to fill time, or something similar.

What specific healthy and appropriate actions have you begun to make a part of your life to address these emotional needs?

_____

_____

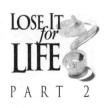

DAY 5:
Forgiveness

In this last lesson for chapter nine of *Lose It for Life*, we want to examine the important role of forgiveness in an all-around healthy, God-honoring lifestyle.

Change is difficult. We all need the help of others and God. Don't be an island determined to do this alone.

Looking at Your *Life*

What is the greatest example of human forgiveness you have ever seen?

_____

_____

Other than God, what person would you say has had to forgive *you* most? Why?

_____

_____

Learning a New Way of *Life*

Jesus said, "For if you forgive men when they sin against you, your heavenly Father will also forgive you. But if you do not forgive men their sins, your Father will not forgive your sins" (Matthew 6:14–15).

What do you think Jesus' words imply?

_____

_____

How does Psalm 66:18 add to your understanding of this passage?

_____

_____

On what occasions did an unforgiving spirit of bitterness toward another person short-circuit the power of God in your life or make Him seem distant?

_____

_____

The authors write: "Forgiveness can be difficult—almost impossible—for those who have been severely abused physically, sexually, and even spiritually. It is never easy or instant, and may take years to complete. However, if forgiveness isn't rendered, the injured person remains trapped in the abuse of the past where they endlessly relive the offenses done against them. Our yesterdays must be put in the past so we can fully enjoy today."

Express your honest reaction to this statement.

_____

_____

Jesus said, "Therefore, if you are offering your gift at the altar and there remember that your brother has something against you, leave your gift there in front of the altar. First go and be reconciled to your brother; then come and offer your gift" (Matthew 5:23–24). In other words, the forgiveness process also involves making things right with those we have wounded. This may require us to write letters or phone calls, to repay debts, to make amends, or otherwise to do our part in making wrongs as right as possible. This, of course, can result in enormous spiritual blessings, both to others and to us.

What people do you need to seek out in order to ask forgiveness? Who did you wrong and how did you wrong them? Be specific. How and when is God urging you to contact them?

_____

_____

Hebrews 12:15 reiterates the need to forgive *everyone* and *anyone* who has hurt you: "Make sure no one gets left out of God's generosity. Keep a sharp eye out for weeds of bitter discontent. A thistle or two gone to seed can ruin a whole garden in no time" (THE MESSAGE).

What are some consequences of becoming bitter and harboring resentment?

_____

_____

Forgiveness, when empowered by God's Spirit, is a process of detaching painful events from our emotional responses to them, thus facilitating the process of healing.

Losing It for *Life*

Forgiveness means:

- handing back our rights to God (the rights we usurped from Him) and inviting Him to be in charge
- asking for forgiveness and making restitution for the damage we've done
- no longer energizing ourselves with rage or hatred
- not trying to change other people, but asking God to do it
- stepping out of the past and into the present
- accepting the pardon of the Cross for others as well as for ourselves
- obeying Jesus' instructions to forgive so that we can be forgiven

Which of the above actions do you find the most difficult to do? Why?

_____

_____

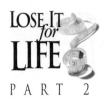

PART 2

"You must make allowance for each other's faults and forgive the person who offends you. Remember, the Lord forgave you, so you must forgive others" (Colossians 3:13 NLT).

Is forgiveness more an emotional state or an act of the will? Why?

_____

_____

If you are aware of anyone at whom you feel intense rage or strong bitterness, what do you intend to do? Why is it imperative that you forgive?

_____

_____

The authors recommend the following prayer:

Dear Lord,
You have commanded me to forgive others, just as you have forgiven me through the sacrifice of your Son, Jesus. I choose to obey You, even though this is not easy for me. You listed all of my sins; then You nailed them to the cross so that Jesus' blood could pay for them. Help me to release this account to You and not seek justice for my sake. Help me to trust that You are just and will carry out whatever punishment is necessary.

Yet, while I transfer this account to You, wounds still remain as a result of this wrong. As I obey You by releasing this person from my debt, I pray that You will heal the hurts they have caused me. Help me to trust that You are willing and able to redeem me from the wrongs that have been done against me. If thoughts of revenge occur, I pray that You will help me continually release this person's account to You. Amen.

Is this a prayer that you need to pray? Make a list here of any slights, grudges, and offenses that you have held on to and would like to release. Then pray about each item, asking the Lord to forgive you (or someone who hurt you) on each point of your list.

_____

_____

In summary, revisit the RISE acronym again. In terms of behavior, we need to:

REDUCE: eating in response to social cues.

INCREASE: the number of changes you make. Start small and add more as you are able.

SUBSTITUTE: forgiveness for any unforgiveness or unresolved misdeed; substitute new behaviors for eating.

ELIMINATE: eating for the wrong reasons.

Preparation: Read chapter ten of Lose It for Life *before you begin the lessons for Week 10.*

DAY 1:
The Miracle and Mystery of Community

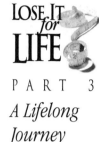

In healthy Christian community we learn to love and be loved, to serve and be served, and to celebrate and be celebrated. In Christian community, we find acceptance, grace, and healing. In Christian community, we hear the truth spoken firmly yet gently, and we learn how to live a new life together. It's no wonder that Lose It For Life believes strongly in the connections made in Christian community. In fact, we do not believe it's possible to live successfully or enjoyably apart from the miracle and mystery of true Christian fellowship.

PART 3

A Lifelong Journey

Here's how to apply the RISE acronym to building community:

REDUCE: negative relationships that sabotage your success.

INCREASE: connection with others; your social skills; your trust in God's ability to turn pain into glory.

SUBSITUTE: the belief that you must go it alone for the understanding that community is a healing gift from God.

ELIMINATE: a lone-ranger mentality and toxic relationships that undermine your success.

We live in a society that values independence, autonomy, and self-sufficiency.

That's what these next five lessons are about.

Looking at Your *Life*

Think back to the closest friendships you ever enjoyed. Maybe it was kids in your neighborhood, a high school team you once played on, a Boy or Girl Scout troop, a collection of roommates, sorority sisters in college, or a small group at church. What made this group of folks and the friendships you enjoyed so meaningful?

_____

_____

_____

Think back to the best church you've ever been a part of. What made it so special?

_____

_____

_____

In your own words, define *community*. Then describe your personal experience of community (whether good or bad) at this point in your life.

_____

_____

_____

PART 3

Learning a New Way of *Life*

Autonomy, individual drive, and self-motivation are admired characteristics in our culture; that is, do it your own way, succeed by your own power. But are these qualities in keeping with the way the body of Christ is designed to function?

Read Genesis 1:26. What do you observe about God in this verse?

_____

_____

_____

Jesus was highly relational. He communed with his heavenly Father, lived and traveled with his disciples, and spent time with all kinds of people.

The authors say: "Relationship is characteristic of the Godhead—they are three in one. The Trinity enjoys fellowship. Relationship has existed from the beginning of time."

In your own words, expand on this idea of God—Father, Son, and Holy Spirit—being in community.

_____

_____

If it's true that we are dependent creatures made in the image of a God who exists "in relationship," what does this suggest about our own needs for community?

_____

_____

_____

Read Acts 2:42–47. Describe the daily lifestyle of the early church. How was their Christian experience different from that of many modern-day churches?

_____

_____

_____

The authors argue:

> If we explore the beginnings of church history in the book of Acts, we find a record of how Christianity was practiced under the power of the Holy Spirit. As the church developed and spread, believers learned to live together, sharing freely with one another while maintaining meaningful fellowship. Even in the face of strong personalities and differences, the church found a way to listen and to submit to one another in Christian love. . . . Through the power of the Holy Spirit and the unity and love practiced in community, believers were healed.

When have you been part of a close-knit fellowship of believers where people cared deeply for one another and actually "did life together" as the early church did? Describe that experience.

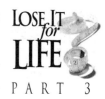

_____

_____

Losing It for *Life*

The New Testament lists a number of attitudes and actions that should mark the lifestyles and interactions of Christians. Here are a few:

> *"A new command I give you: Love one another. As I have loved you, so you must love one another. By this all men will know that you are my disciples, if you love one another"* (John 13:34–35).

> *"Honor one another above yourselves"* (Romans 12:10).

> *"Live in harmony with one another"* (Romans 12:16).

> *"Therefore let us stop passing judgment on one another"* (Romans 14:13).

> *"Accept one another, then, just as Christ accepted you, in order to bring praise to God"* (Romans 15:7).

> *"I appeal to you, brothers, in the name of our Lord Jesus Christ, that all of you agree with one another so that there may be no divisions among you and that you may be perfectly united in mind and thought"* (1 Corinthians 1:10).

> *"Be kind and compassionate to one another, forgiving each other, just as in Christ God forgave you"* (Ephesians 4:32).

In what specific ways does living by these "one another" commands build healthier, happier community?

_____

_____

How effectively does your church live by these commands?

_____

_____

Go back through the list and grade yourself. Which of these "one anothers" are you faithful to put into practice on a regular basis?

_____

_____

_____

LOSE IT for LIFE

PART 3

Relationships are necessary to meet our needs for intimacy and to help us grow and avoid relapse into old, unhealthy lifestyle habits.

Which of these commands have you been guilty of neglecting? In what areas do you need improvement?

_____

_____

What new thing did you learn about community from this lesson? Or, what old truth were you reminded to put into practice today?

_____

_____

_____

DAY 2:
Overeating versus Community

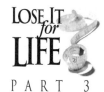

PART 3

Perhaps you've never thought about it, but overeating and weight problems can disconnect us from one another. In this lesson we want to explore how unhealthy eating habits often contribute to dysfunctional relationships, and, on the other hand, how healthy eating habits can be encouraged by functional relationships/community.

When we are obsessed with food and weight, we often hide or pull back from active involvement with others.

Looking at Your *Life*

How do you feel when overweight people are made fun of on television programs or by comedians?

_____

_____

If you have ever been made to feel like a social outcast because of your weight, what happened in your heart? How did the experience alter the way you related to people?

_____

_____

If you have ever been bullied or verbally abused because of your weight, write some candid memories of those experiences.

_____

_____

What people have accepted you with no strings attached—fully and completely, despite your weight or appearance?

_____

_____

What can you do to express your appreciation to those folks?

_____

_____

Learning a New Way of *Life*

Take a few minutes to read through the entire prayer that Jesus prayed in John 17. Then focus on this excerpt:

> *"My prayer is not for [the twelve apostles] alone. I pray also for those who will believe in me through their message [Christians down through the centuries—including us!]*

177

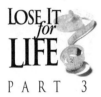

PART 3

that all of them may be one, Father, just as you are in me and I am in you. May they also be in us so that the world may believe that you have sent me. I have given them the glory that you gave me, that they may be one as we are one: I in them and you in me. May they be brought to complete unity to let the world know that you sent me and have loved them even as you have loved me." (John 17:20–23,bracketed material added)

How would you summarize the main point of Jesus' prayer? What is it that He wants for the world? For His followers?

_____

_____

How do you think our enemy, the devil, might view Christian unity and healthy community?

_____

_____

When we pull back from others and remain isolated and alone because of our weight (or for any other reason), how do you think God feels about it?

_____

_____

Consider these situations and offer your assessment, based on what you just studied.

Situation...	What God might think/feel	How Satan probably reacts
You resist an invitation to a ski party at the lake because of your weight.		
You take lunch early and eat by yourself in your car rather than with colleagues.		
You tell yourself you'll become more sociable when you drop about 50 pounds.		
You drop out of a small group because someone told a "fat" joke.		
You come late to social events and leave early if food is involved.		

Look again at Romans 15:7. This verse stresses the importance of accepting others. What other important fact does it reveal about Christ? How does that truth help us build a healthier self-image?

_____

_____

The authors point out that when someone loses a large amount of weight, one of the common expectations is that life will be dramatically better. The reasoning goes like this: *When I lose weight, I'll get lots of invitations and everything will be different. Socially, I'll become outgoing and active.*

But then, they point out, the weight comes off and reality hits. *Where are all those new party invitations? Why don't people see the new me and invite me out?*

This happens because an overweight person learns to feel uneasy in social situations. He or she develops deeply-ingrained habits of hiding, avoiding, and withdrawing. Just because a person's body is getting thinner doesn't mean that his or her heart is now oozing with courage and confidence. Losing weight does not automatically result in losing fears of rejection. We still have to take social and relational risks.

React to this statement: "The inside of a person can still struggle with major insecurities even when the outside is looking healthier."

_____

_____

_____

Losing It for *Life*

How can and should you respond to people who are not positive and affirming?

_____

_____

How does knowing—deep in your soul—that Christ accepts and loves you unconditionally make a difference in your effort to become healthier physically, emotionally, socially, and spiritually?

_____

_____

On whom can you count for faithful support and encouragement?

_____

_____

LOSE IT
for
LIFE

PART 3

Regardless of what you weigh, it's up to you to push yourself out there in the unpredictable world of relationships.

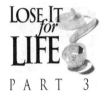

PART 3

The authors observe: "When you are the consummate giver and never expect to receive in a relationship, you tend to attract needy people who can suck you dry. And then, guess what? You feel empty and use food to fill that void again." Have you experienced this in your life? Explain.

_____

_____

Community is so important. When you feel strong, you encourage others. When you are down, others support you. This reciprocal give-and-take is part of healthy relationships.

Do you feel comfortable "needing" others? Are you more at ease giving or taking?

_____

_____

In Day 1 you read through several New Testament "one another" commands (guidelines for healthy community). Here are a few more to ponder and put into practice:

"Speak to one another with psalms, hymns and spiritual songs" (Ephesians 5:19).

"Submit to one another out of reverence for Christ" (Ephesians 5:21).

"Therefore encourage one another and build each other up, just as in fact you are doing" (1 Thessalonians 5:11).

"And let us consider how we may spur one another on toward love and good deeds" (Hebrews 10:24).

"Offer hospitality to one another without grumbling" (1 Peter 4:9).

"All of you, clothe yourselves with humility toward one another, because, 'God opposes the proud but gives grace to the humble'" (1 Peter 5:5).

How can living out these commands and associating with others who hold these values make a difference in losing it for life?

_____

_____

DAY 3:
Social Skills

Weight loss may boost your confidence in how you look but it won't teach you how to interact with others. In this lesson we'll focus on social skills—changing for the better the way you interact with others.

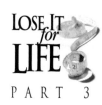

LOSE IT *for* LIFE

PART 3

Looking at Your *Life*

How sociable are you? How good are your skills at relating to others? Rate yourself on a continuum of 1–10 in the following areas.

1= low (I need improvement); 10 = high (I do this really well)

Social skills must be practiced. If you've spent a lifetime hiding, you may have to practice new skills.

	1	2	3	4	5	6	7	8	9	10
Smiling at others										
Making eye contact										
Feeling at ease around people										
Taking the initiative to speak										
Making conversation										
Making others feel comfortable										
Making others feel cared for										
Making people feel included										
Listening										
Drawing people out										
Showing hospitality										
Showing compassion										
Being assertive										
Gathering people										
Displaying a sense of humor										

What areas received your lowest marks? Why did you give yourself these low scores?

_____

_____

Who do you know that displays ease and grace in social settings? What do you think is their secret?

_____

_____

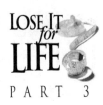

PART 3

If you are tired of no social life, then begin to create one.

Learning a New Way of *Life*

Reflect on the following Scripture passages:

"Do to others as you would have them do to you" (Luke 6:31).

"Do nothing out of selfish ambition or vain conceit, but in humility consider others better than yourselves. Each of you should look not only to your own interests, but also to the interests of others. Your attitude should be the same as that of Christ Jesus" (Philippians 2:3–5).

"Be devoted to one another in brotherly love. Honor one another above yourselves" (Romans 12:10).

What do these verses suggest about the way we are called by God to relate to others?

_____

_____

Why is hanging back and avoiding others not an option for those who claim to be followers of Christ?

_____

_____

_____

After reading chapter ten of *Lose It for Life,* imagine that a reclusive friend of yours says, "Look—I'm just shy. That's the way I am and the way I've always been. I can't help that. God made me with this personality. I feel like all this emphasis on 'social skills' is an attempt to make me become something I'm not." What would you say? Is this a legitimate argument?

_____

_____

Just the thought of doing something new (for example, taking social risks) can be nerve-wracking. If you are anxious about taking some new risks, think about Jesus' words: "Peace I leave with you; my peace I give you. I do not give to you as the world gives. Do not let your hearts be troubled and do not be afraid" (John 14:27). How does this promise help you?

_____

_____

How do we access this supernatural peace and banish our fears of rejection?

_____

_____

Losing It for *Life*

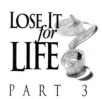

The LIFL book suggests a few practical ways to get out there mixing and mingling with others. One suggestion: "Today, make it your goal to approach someone you would like to get to know better. Find out an interest he or she has and begin to ask about it."

Jot down your honest reaction to that recommendation.

_____

_____

How much do the following beliefs or attitudes contribute to your own reluctance to engage others?

	A LOT	**SOME**	**BARELY AT ALL**
I have nothing to offer.			
I'm ugly and unworthy.			
I'm afraid of rejection.			
I never know what to do or say.			
I'm okay. I really don't need others.			
I've been hurt before—never again.			
People are fickle/untrustworthy.			
I'll just embarrass myself.			
People take advantage of me.			
I feel awkward and just freeze up.			

Which of these attitudes do you want to begin working on? What's your specific plan to address this area of needed change?

_____

_____

In the book we read: "Yet even with all our reasons for pulling back and protecting ourselves from hurt or pain, we still desire connection. We were created to relate to God and others. It is in relationships we grow and learn about ourselves. Through our experiences with others we define how we think and feel. Attachment is a basic need that never goes away but longs to be met. And while we try to meet that need through eating, the need is never satisfied."

LOSE IT for LIFE
PART 3

When we are willing to be open, transparent, and vulnerable with others, we break the isolation that has kept us hidden and in the dark.

Your comments, thoughts, reaction? How do you handle the ambivalence of wanting connection and fearing it?

_____

_____

Relationships contain risks, but they also contain rewards. How can we overcome our fear of the former so that we boldly pursue the latter?

_____

_____

Think about the relationships in your life right now. Do you need more? Do you want deeper connection with others? Or do you want to stay on the same path you're on?

_____

_____

Remember, you are on a certain life trajectory. In other words, your current habits and ways of thinking and relating have you pointed in a certain direction that leads to a final destination.

As you fast-forward your life, is that destination the place you really want to end up? Or, would you like a different outcome?

_____

_____

It's pretty basic. The only way to end up in a different place is to go in a new direction. That means making little changes today.

What social interaction changes do you intend to make beginning today? (Be specific: "I'm going to walk over to Debbie's cubicle at work, smile, and tell her good morning." Or "I'm going to ask Debbie if she wants to go with me to lunch.") Make your list in this space. Write at least three clear, measurable, achievable social goals.

_____

_____

_____

_____

DAY 4:
Sabotage!

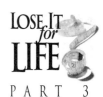

P A R T   3

How many times have you or someone you know complained that they lacked any real support for weight loss? It's a fact: those around us and in our intimate relationships can actually block or sabotage our efforts! That's the focus of this lesson.

Looking at Your *Life*

If you are married, have you ever felt that your spouse was unsupportive of your attempts to lose weight? What do you think might be the reason?

_____

_____

The authors write: "In some cases, husbands worry that their wives' thinner appearances will make them more vulnerable to other men. In other cases, if one spouse takes responsibility for a weight problem, there may be the expectation that the other spouse tackle a specific problem like anger, drinking, or gambling."

Do these worries seem like a legitimate possibility?

_____

_____

_____

What has happened when you have tried to get your spouse to go on a diet, to exercise, or to lose weight with you?

_____

_____

When has a spouse/boyfriend or girlfriend/parent ever demanded that you lose weight? How did that make you feel?

_____

_____

How do you typically respond when people *demand* a certain behavior from you?

_____

_____

_____

Weight loss efforts can also be sabotaged because you've spent your life being a "victim." To move out of the victim role means forgiving people and making changes.

185

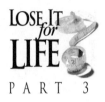

Learning a New Way of *Life*

Whenever we begin to change, it affects everyone around us. People are used to the old you. But now you're eating differently, exercising regularly, processing your "stuff," changing your attitudes. You're becoming more honest, more vulnerable, and more outgoing. All these things are good and God-honoring, but that doesn't mean your LIFL experience will always be easy and positive. You'll have times of frustration and you'll learn who can handle your new way of thinking and living and who cannot.

Avoiding these new conflicts means either, (a) avoiding people altogether—*not* an option, as we've already seen, or (b) learning better how to cultivate good relationships and live in harmony with those who don't always agree with you.

Consider this passage from Romans 14 that touches on that very subject:

> *"Welcome with open arms fellow believers who don't see things the way you do. And don't jump all over them every time they do or say something you don't agree with—even when it seems that they are strong on opinions but weak in the faith department. Remember, they have their own history to deal with. Treat them gently.*
>
> *For instance, a person who has been around for a while might well be convinced that he can eat anything on the table, while another, with a different background, might assume all Christians should be vegetarians and eat accordingly. But since both are guests at Christ's table, wouldn't it be terribly rude if they fell to criticizing what the other ate or didn't eat? God, after all, invited them both to the table. Do you have any business crossing people off the guest list or interfering with God's welcome? If there are corrections to be made or manners to be learned, God can handle that without your help.*
>
> *Or, say, one person thinks that some days should be set aside as holy and another thinks that each day is pretty much like any other. There are good reasons either way. So, each person is free to follow the convictions of conscience. What's important in all this is that if you keep a holy day, keep it for God's sake; if you eat meat, eat it to the glory of God and thank God for prime rib; if you're a vegetarian, eat vegetables to the glory of God and thank God for broccoli.*
>
> *None of us are permitted to insist on our own way in these matters. It's God we are answerable to—all the way from life to death and everything in between—not each other. That's why Jesus lived and died and then lived again: so that he could be our Master across the entire range of life and death, and free us from the petty tyrannies of each other"* (THE MESSAGE).

How do Paul's words of counsel speak to your LIFL experience?

_____

_____

How exactly does Jesus "free us from the petty tyrannies of each other"? Give examples from your own life.

_____

_____

Ephesians 4:2 says, "Be completely humble and gentle; be patient, bearing with one another in love." How would compliance with this command make a tangible difference in your closest relationships?

_____

_____

You can't change others, but you can—with God's help—change your own attitudes and behavior. If you are guilty of pride and harshness and impatience, what do you need to do to correct things?

_____

_____

The authors argue that relationships are work because they often act as mirrors to our own problems. It's when we're close to others that we most vividly see our own shortcomings and our need for God's help. As we mature, we become aware of our uniqueness and also our need for others. We learn to define who we are, set boundaries, deal with conflict, appreciate and manage differences, *but only so long as we stay connected to others in the process.*

What do you like about this observation? What about it is difficult for you?

_____

_____

Losing It for *Life*

Studies show that spousal support and the support of families and other friends is very important when it comes to losing weight.[1]

Did you have any good, substantive discussions of your goals with others before beginning the LIFL program? It may be helpful now to think through or discuss with someone your hidden fears or concerns about your losing weight. (Remember: The best situation is when your intimate relationships can be part of your support system!)

Galatians 5:22–23 describes the things that build healthy relationships in our lives: "But the fruit of the [Holy] Spirit [the work which His presence within accomplishes] is love, joy (gladness), peace, patience (an even temper, forbearance), kindness, goodness (benevolence), faithfulness, gentleness (meekness, humility), self-control (self-restraint, continence). Against such things there is no law [that can bring a charge]" (AMP).

LOSE IT
for
LIFE

PART 3

Relationships make the difference in your ability to survive and come through trials. Have the courage to stay in relationships with others.

187

LOSE IT
for
LIFE
PART 3

Articles posted on the LIFL website can help you get started and encourage you to keep "losing and moving for life."

What evidence of the fruit of the Holy Spirit do you see in your current dealings with other people?

_____

_____

_____

LIFL counselors online at the LIFL website (www.loseitforlife.com) can be a helpful resource, and will offer on-going support. You can ask them questions any time. On-going interaction and accountability may be just what is needed to get you moving forward for life!

Have you accessed this help on the web? How about the message board on the LIFL website? Or have you visited the Online Community in the Chat Room to talk about your victories and struggles? In what ways can this support help in your journey?

_____

_____

_____

What do you think of the suggestion of taking some social risks and starting your own LIFL group? Think about it—you could gather together some friends or fellow strugglers and form a support group in your community. Use this book and print additional materials from the Online Community to use in a group setting. Groups are great ways to encourage one another and hold each other accountable. What's holding you back? What steps can you take to starting a group?

_____

_____

DAY 5:
Trading Your Pain for His Purposes

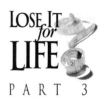

PART 3

The Bible says that God comes alongside us when we go through difficulty. That in and of itself is reassuring, but there is even more—God wants to use us to help others who are going through a hard time. In God's economy, nothing is ever wasted, not even our pain. In this final lesson from week 10, we'll do a quick study of what's involved in trading our pain for God's purposes.

The Christian gospel brings a profound promise of evil being transformed into eternal good, weakness into strength, and tragedy into triumph.

Looking at Your *Life*

When you were a child, what was your favorite fairy tale? What did you like about it?

_____

_____

_____

Why are fairy tales so popular?

_____

_____

_____

_____

In what ways is real life *different* from fairy tales? In what ways is it *similar*?

_____

_____

_____

_____

Is "happily ever after" a foolish dream? Or for the Christian, is it the way God works?

_____

_____

_____

_____

What tough or even tragic incidents can you remember in your life that ultimately led to something good?

_____

_____

_____

Learning a New Way of *Life*

LOSE IT for LIFE

PART 3

What is your typical reaction to hard or unpleasant trials? (Check all that apply)

_____ I pout.

_____ I cry.

_____ I scream and yell.

_____ I eat.

_____ I look for distractions.

_____ I throw things.

_____ I curse.

_____ I thank God.

_____ I trust that God has his reasons.

_____ I clam up.

_____ I pray.

_____ I complain.

_____ I get angry.

_____ I laugh (so that I don't cry).

_____ I try not to think about it.

_____ I quote my favorite Bible verses.

_____ I call my friends.

_____ Other (specify):

Second Corinthians 1:3–4 says: "All praise to the God and Father of our Master, Jesus the Messiah! Father of all mercy! God of all healing counsel! He comes alongside us when we go through hard times, and before you know it, he brings us alongside someone else who is going through hard times so that we can be there for that person just as God was there for us" (THE MESSAGE).

What does this passage promise?

_____

_____

Share a personal example for each of the following truths about trials:

- "We can never know God's plans, glorify Him, or accept His gain from our loss, unless we give Him our misery."

_____

_____

- "Once our loss and pain point us to God's grace, we can also lead others into His grace."

LOSE IT
for
LIFE

PART 3

_____

_____

_____

_____

In 2 Corinthians 4:16–17 we read, "Therefore we do not lose heart. Though outwardly we are wasting away, yet inwardly we are being renewed day by day. For our light and momentary troubles are achieving for us an eternal glory that far outweighs them all."

What different perspective does this passage offer regarding difficulties and trials?

_____

_____

_____

_____

_____

God's ultimate goal for us is nothing less than total transformation. Second Corinthians 3:18 says, "As the Spirit of the Lord works within us, we become more and more like him and reflect his glory even more" (NLT).

Don't you want God to take your years of struggle with weight problems and transform it all for His glory? If so, you will emerge from this experience stronger and more able to help others along the way.

Look at the following "Transformation Report Card." Evaluate yourself with A–F.

_____ Learning how to forgive others (and doing it!)

_____ Loving others unselfishly and deeply

_____ Being honest with God and others about who I am

_____ Becoming aware of my spiritual gifts

_____ Carrying the message of spiritual transformation to others

_____ Reaching out in compassion to those facing similar struggles to our own

_____ Surrendering to the truth that God is working all things together for good

_____ Seeking to apply past pain to positive purposes

_____ No longer saying, Why me, Lord?" but saying instead, "What do you want me to learn and do here?"

_____ Being a giver instead of a taker

_____ Learning to listen rather than always needing to be heard

_____ Allowing humbling experiences to give me a servant's heart

_____ Investing my spiritual gifts in the lives of others

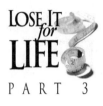

PART 3

Losing It for *Life*

Training is hard work, but the payoff feels so good. We are all in training for the eternal, and what we do today matters.

How does serious, sometimes agonizing training help athletes? How can serious spiritual training help us?

_____

_____

_____

What happens if we give up at the first signs of difficulty?

_____

_____

_____

What practical steps can we take to become tougher and more resilient in the face of tough times?

_____

_____

_____

List six things (biblical truths, people, goals, etc.) that you can lean on this next month to help you stay in the Lose It For Life race.

_____

_____

_____

Here's a prayer for endurance. If it expresses your desire, voice it to God. Or write your own prayer.

Heavenly Father,
When I feel like giving up, when I think I can't go on, give me strong reminders of your love and help. You desire for me to go the distance. Your reward is great, both today and eternally. Help me to keep my eyes fixed on You and the final prize. Give me the strength to endure when I think I can't. Amen.

Preparation: Read chapter eleven of Lose It for Life *before you begin the lessons for Week 11.*

DAY 1:
The Danger of Relapse

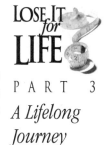

PART 3

A Lifelong Journey

By now you know that *Losing It for Life* is not something you do quickly or half-heartedly. You are engaged in a lifelong, 24/7, comprehensive, external, *and* internal transformation. Always lurking is the danger of losing heart, losing your way, retreating. How to guard against that possibility is the focus of these final lessons.

Looking at Your *Life*

Take a self-inventory test. Check all the following statements that are true of you.

_____ I like to visit the places I lived as a child.

_____ I go to reunions (class, family, and others) whenever I can.

_____ People say I am nostalgic.

_____ Unlike many people, I actually watch my old home videos from time to time.

_____ I enjoy television re-runs.

_____ I tell lots of stories from my childhood.

_____ I often fail to learn from my mistakes.

_____ I prefer music from my younger days.

_____ I watch my favorite movies over and over.

_____ I pull out old picture albums periodically and enjoy looking back.

_____ I think about the past as much or more as I think about the future.

What, if anything, does this exercise reveal about yourself?

_____

_____

_____

Describe three life events you'd love to go back and experience again.

_____

_____

Describe three experiences you'd rather not repeat—*ever*.

_____

_____

_____

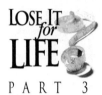

LOSE IT for LIFE

PART 3

The authors remind us that we can know what to do and be doing it, and yet still slip back into old patterns of behavior, thinking, and feeling. What are your biggest fears about your weight loss and keeping it off?

_____

_____

_____

Whenever you deal with a chronic problem like weight loss, you have to be willing to do whatever it takes to avoid relapse.

Learning a New Way of *Life*

Writing about his struggle to know and serve Christ, the apostle Paul described his resolve to keep pressing ahead and not give up:

> *"Not that I have already obtained all this, or have already been made perfect, but I press on to take hold of that for which Christ Jesus took hold of me. Brothers, I do not consider myself yet to have taken hold of it. But one thing I do: Forgetting what is behind and straining toward what is ahead, I press on toward the goal to win the prize for which God has called me heavenward in Christ Jesus" (Philippians 3:12–14).*

Go through that passage carefully and circle the verbs. What kind of action do they describe?

_____

_____

Of all the disciples chosen by Christ, Peter seemed the most solid and the most dependable. He even earned the name, "Rock." It was Peter, speaking for all the rest, who confidently and correctly answered the ultimate question about Jesus' true identity. "You are the Christ," he declared, "the Son of the Living God" (Matthew 16:16).

Then, after three years of listening to Jesus and following Him, after hearing life-changing words and witnessing jaw-dropping miracles, Peter received a sobering warning from the Lord about failing and falling (Luke 22:31–34). Peter was shocked—even wounded. He protested loudly. "Not me!" he insisted. "Never!"

Read Luke 22:54–62. What does Peter's experience teach you?

_____

_____

How have you recently wrestled with having "good intentions" but not keeping them?

_____

_____

Losing It for *Life*

Good intentions are not enough against great temptations. Planning is key to preventing relapse. You have to begin recovery and follow through, or you place yourself at risk for relapse. We want you to be successful losing weight and keeping it off. So let's concentrate on preventing relapse.

Define *relapse* in your own terms.

_____

_____

Relapse is more than a "slip" or return to overeating. It involves a predictable progression until, ultimately, you revert to old patterns.

What's the difference between "slipping" in the area of eating, and a full-fledged relapse?

_____

_____

Describe a "driftwood" approach to eating/weight loss/exercise/etc.

_____

_____

Describe a "piloted sailboat" approach to eating/weight loss/exercise/etc.

_____

_____

What time of day, or what day of the week, or in what situations are you most tempted to give up and say, "I'm just gonna live my comfortable old life"?

_____

_____

How much do feelings of failure, self-disgust, or hopelessness contribute to people's relapsing into old patterns? What do you think is the solution to these negative thoughts and feelings?

_____

_____

Identify one or two helpful conclusions from this lesson that can you tuck away in your mental "Relapse Response Kit."

_____

_____

_____

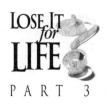

LOSE IT
for
LIFE
PART 3

Planning is key to preventing relapse.

DAY 2:
Signs of Relapse

If you can recognize the signs of relapse early, you will know when you are moving into dangerous waters and you can choose to get back on track.

Looking at Your *Life*

Relate the idea of recognizing early warning signs to other areas of your life. Look at the following areas. Write out what specific early warning signs you might see that would prompt you to take action. . . .

• where your child's academic performance is involved?

_____

_____

_____

• where your vehicle is concerned?

_____

_____

• with regard to your financial condition?

_____

_____

_____

• regarding the health of your marriage?

_____

_____

_____

• in the area of your own medical health?

_____

_____

_____

• concerning a parent's ability to live independently?

_____

_____

_____

What safeguards do you have in place to alert you to potential trouble in your LIFL journey? (For example, "My scales—when my weight hits _____ lbs., I know something is wrong.")

_____

_____

_____

Learning a New Way of *Life*

Many people who followed Jesus for a while found His teachings too difficult to put into practice and eventually stopped following Him. They came face-to-face with ultimate truth and turned away.

What do you think prompts reasonably smart people to reject the very things that can rescue them?

_____

_____

_____

The apostle Paul urged: "If you think you are standing strong, be careful, for you, too, may fall into the same sin" (1 Corinthians 10:12 NLT). In what ways is this verse timeless advice for many areas of life?

_____

_____

When things are going well, why do we tend to drop our guard and become vulnerable to failure? Cite examples of this from your life (not necessarily pertaining to weight loss).

_____

_____

Read the following warnings from Scripture:

> *And pray in the Spirit on all occasions with all kinds of prayers and requests. With this in mind, be alert and always keep on praying for all the saints. (Ephesians 6:18)*

> *So then, let us not be like others, who are asleep, but let us be alert and self-controlled. (1 Thessalonians 5:6)*

> *Be self-controlled and alert. Your enemy the devil prowls around like a roaring lion looking for someone to devour. (1 Peter 5:8)*

How do these truths apply to your LIFL program?

_____

_____

LOSE IT for LIFE

PART 3

Each new struggle or obstacle presents us with a choice: We can cave in and quit. Or we can lean hard into God, letting Him fill us with new strength.

197

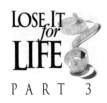

Losing It for *Life*

Based on much research and experience, we've identified common thoughts, feelings, and behaviors that are warning signs for relapse. Read through the chart, then work through the accompanying questions.

PART 3

When I start *feeling*...	I begin *thinking*...	What I *do* is...	I *become*...
Victimized & entitled	Not my fault; others are to blame	Lie & present a false self	Dishonest
Sorry for myself; resentful & depressed	The world owes me & revolves around me	Anything I want; have a "pity party"	Negative, self-centered
Irritated, impatient, dissatisfied	"I need it NOW...this is taking too long"	Get impulsive and argue a lot	Intolerant, easily frustrated
Stressed & worried; fearful	In confused and indecisive ways	Become paralyzed (and fail to follow a plan)	Anxious
Over-confident, powerful, arrogant	"I'm the exception to the rule. I've got it made. I'll show them. I'll be the center of attention."	Play counselor, impress others with my accomplishments, be generous to a fault	Grandiose
Guilty over never doing enough and driven to do more	Nothing is ever right. "I must make up for past mistakes."	Cut myself off from others	Perfectionistic
Fearful of the future; regretful of the past	If only ... (fantasizing excessively)	Live according to "shoulds" and not needs	Trapped in a "there & then" mindset / way of life
Conflicted internally	"No one knows but me"	Run from help; express destructive feelings; rebel	Defiant
Bored; lonely	"I don't belong ... I don't need anyone ... I can do it myself... No one cares."	Withdraw; reject help	Isolated; disconnected

Which situations in the chart do you most readily identify with?

_____

_____

Which feelings are most common? Which thoughts are a regular part of your mindset?

_____

_____

What connection do you see between what we think and feel and what we do?

_____

_____

_____

Go back through the chart and see if you can explain how the elements in each row (thoughts, emotions) can logically lead to overeating.

Look at the last column—which of those words or phrases typically describe you. What do you want to do about that? What words would you prefer others used to describe your personality/character?

_____

_____

_____

LOSE IT
for
LIFE

P A R T   3

A prayer of Jeremiah the prophet: "O Lord, you alone can heal me; you alone can save. My praises are for you alone!" (Jeremiah 17:14 NLT)

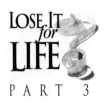

DAY 3:
Phases of Relapse

Because relapse is a gradual process building over time, you should be aware of the phases of relapse as well. This lesson can help.

Looking at Your *Life*

Describe what dynamics are going on in each of the following scenarios.

- You're at the beach. The sand, the water, and the weather—it's all glorious. You get on a floating raft in the warm aquamarine waves out in front of your hotel. You are so relaxed that you doze off. When you awake 35 minutes later you realize that your hotel *moved!* It's 500 yards down the beach!

_____

_____

- You normally run a tight ship at home—everything spotless and in order and highly organized. Last month, however, was *crazy*. A family medical mini-crisis, a huge musical/drama production at church, kids playing on two sports teams in two different leagues, several quick out-of-town trips, plus you've been nursing a really painful lower back. You wake up one Saturday morning, and notice—for the first time in weeks— how dirty and messy your home is. Why it looks almost like a frat house!

_____

_____

- Six months ago you were extremely passionate about your faith. You had something of a spiritual awakening and couldn't get enough of God. You devoured the Bible and looked forward to small group meetings like a kid looks forward to Christmas. Now, for some reason, you feel blah, ho-hum, disinterested. The Bible seems dry and irrelevant.

_____

_____

_____

The Second Law of Thermodynamics basically says that things tend toward disorder. What examples have you experienced in your own life? If this law is true, what is the solution? How can we avoid losing the gains we've made?

_____

_____

Learning a New Way of *Life*

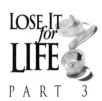

We must be proactive in watching for relapse. It's easy to drift along. The story of David's adultery with Bathsheba is a case study in how we can gradually end up in places where we don't want to be.

Read 2 Samuel 11, and note the foolish choices David made along the way.

_____

_____

_____

Demas was a Christian brother mentioned in some of Paul's epistles. The final mention of him is rather solemn: "Demas, because he loved this world, has deserted me and has gone to Thessalonica" (2 Timothy 4:10).

"We must pay more careful attention, therefore, to what we have heard, so that we do not drift away" (Hebrews 2:1).

What do you suppose happened? What might have been in Thessalonica that caused Demas to chuck everything?

_____

_____

_____

Why do you suppose God included this "cautionary tale" in His Word?

_____

_____

_____

King Solomon had some huge advantages. He had a godly father, whom the Bible describes as a man after God's own heart (see Acts 13:22); he was given an infusion of supernatural wisdom (1 Kings 3:5–15) and the promise of God's presence and protection if he remained faithful to God (1 Kings 9).

Read 1 Kings 11. What happened?

_____

_____

_____

What's the lesson for us?

_____

_____

_____

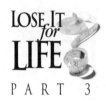

LOSE IT for LIFE

PART 3

Losing It for *Life*

Review the stages of relapse below, and see how much you know about what to do to ward off each danger.

• Complacency

What is it? _____

What causes it? _____

What does it look like in *your* life? _____

How can you combat it? _____

• Confusion

What is it? _____

What causes it? _____

What does it look like in *your* life? _____

How can you combat it? _____

• Compromise

What is it? _____

What causes it? _____

What does it look like in *your* life? _____

How can you combat it? _____

• Catastrophe

What is it? _____

What causes it? _____

What does it look like in *your* life? _____

How can you combat it? _____

DAY 4:
Protection from Relapse

In order to prevent relapse, you need to establish a system of protection. That is the focus of this workbook lesson.

Looking at Your *Life*

Which of the following kinds of daily protection do you have or do you use?

- ❏ Computer virus protection software
- ❏ Internet filters
- ❏ smoke alarms
- ❏ water purification system
- ❏ burglar alarm system
- ❏ vehicle anti-theft device
- ❏ sunscreen with high SPF
- ❏ child safety latches on your cabinets
- ❏ safety deposit box
- ❏ surge protectors on sensitive electronics

What kind of protections—emotionally, spiritually, or physically—do you have in place to help you avoid a relapse?

_____

_____

_____

We're nearing the end of this LIFL workbook, so let's assess a few things.

What specific, identifiable changes have you made since beginning this new adventure? List at least ten.

_____

_____

_____

What's proving more difficult for you—cutting out certain eating habits or adding exercise routines?

_____

_____

"Do not withhold your mercy from me, O LORD; may your love and your truth always protect me" (Psalms 40:11).

LOSE IT for LIFE

PART 3

LOSE IT
for
LIFE
PART 3

What has been the single most helpful insight you've gained? You're biggest "aha!" revelation?

_____

_____

_____

_____

"May the Lord direct your hearts into God's love and Christ's perseverance" (2 Thessalonians 3:5).

Learning a New Way of *Life*

Remember the Old Testament story of Caleb? Caleb and Joshua boldly (but unsuccessfully) urged the Israelites to trust God and conquer their enemies inhabiting the Promised Land. Because of the people's stubbornness and lack of faith, Caleb spent almost half of his life trudging through a desert wasteland.

Then God gave His people a second opportunity to conquer Canaan. Caleb could have said, "Look, I've done enough already. I fought hard and tried my best once before. And look where it got me. Quite frankly, I'm tired. Why struggle day after day? No thanks. I think I'll kick back and live off the memory of that one shining moment when I really went for it." But he didn't. Instead, here's what happened:

> *"Now the men of Judah approached Joshua at Gilgal, and Caleb son of Jephunneh the Kenizzite said to him, 'You know what the LORD said to Moses the man of God at Kadesh Barnea about you and me. I was forty years old when Moses the servant of the LORD sent me from Kadesh Barnea to explore the land. And I brought him back a report according to my convictions, but my brothers who went up with me made the hearts of the people melt with fear. I, however, followed the LORD my God wholeheartedly. So on that day Moses swore to me, "The land on which your feet have walked will be your inheritance and that of your children forever, because you have followed the LORD my God wholeheartedly."*
>
> *Now then, just as the LORD promised, he has kept me alive for forty-five years since the time he said this to Moses, while Israel moved about in the desert. So here I am today, eighty-five years old! I am still as strong today as the day Moses sent me out; I'm just as vigorous to go out to battle now as I was then. Now give me this hill country that the LORD promised me that day. You yourself heard then that the Anakites were there and their cities were large and fortified, but, the LORD helping me, I will drive them out just as he said'" (Joshua 14:6–12).*

Put yourself in Caleb's sandals. How would you have responded?

_____

_____

_____

_____

What qualities did Caleb have that you admire?

_____

_____

_____

_____

How does a person develop these virtues?

_____

_____

_____

_____

LOSE IT
for
LIFE

P A R T   3

Avoid "if-only" thinking. It is not compatible with surrender; instead it reflects an attitude of discontent.

Losing It for *Life*

In chapter eleven of the LIFL book is a list of a number of protections we can build into our lives to avoid relapse. Let's review them and think about them in more detail.

The authors write: "Exercise and physical activity are essential to a healthy lifestyle and must be a part of your regular, daily routine." How is your plan/program to "get your body moving" coming along? What types of activity have you settled on as most suited for you?

_____

_____

_____

_____

Do you think you've made the switch from viewing your changes in eating as a "temporary diet" to a "whole new way of life"? Why or why not?

_____

_____

_____

_____

How can rest and relaxation protect against relapse? What are your favorite replenishing activities?

_____

_____

_____

LOSE IT for LIFE

PART 3

A huge premise of the LIFL plan is that lasting external change requires a solid internal foundation. What specific steps have you taken to help you develop and maintain a steady, healthy relationship with God? What spiritual disciplines have you incorporated into your regular lifestyle?

_____

_____

_____

What's the wisdom in living "one day at a time" (Matthew 6:34)?

_____

_____

_____

We've talked about it at length, but how does accountability provide a safety net? List your sources of accountability.

_____

_____

_____

DAY 5:
Preserving Our Gains and Moving On

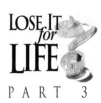

Congratulations! You've done it. You've made it to the end of this workbook. Of course, that doesn't mean the work is done. Losing It For Life is a lifestyle, not a short-term project or experiment. But the good news is that you now are armed with information you didn't have a short time ago.

With God's help, you've begun implementing new strategies and plans that really *do* have the potential to enable you to live in freedom and joy. Let's spend this last section celebrating and remembering a few crucial details.

With God, it's possible to lose it for life and keep it off. To Him be the glory!

Looking at Your *Life*

The word *mediocre* comes from two Latin words, *media*, meaning "in the middle of," and *ocris*, meaning "mountain." Literally then, to be *mediocre* is to be "midway up the mountain." Perhaps the picture is of a mountain climber who starts out with grand ambitions and big dreams, but who then gets weary during the arduous ascent. Stopping on a ledge to catch his breath, the climber stops focusing on where he still wants to go. Instead, he looks back down at how far he has come and begins to become self-satisfied, complacent. As a result, rather than pressing on for the summit, he settles in. He has become *mediocre*.

Thinking back, what are some areas where you've been tempted to become mediocre and settle, saying, "Well, it isn't what I originally hoped for, but I guess it's good enough"?

_____

_____

_____

_____

Define *excellence*. How does it require an ever-increasing commitment to make progress?

_____

_____

_____

_____

What part of this program that you have studied and implemented encourages you the most right now?

_____

_____

_____

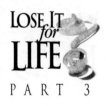

PART 3

But thanks be to God! He gives us the victory through our Lord Jesus Christ (1 Corinthians 15:57).

Learning a New Way of *Life*

The apostle Paul's letter to the Colossian Christians begins with a glorious tribute to Jesus Christ. Notice how He is described:

"He is the image of the invisible God, the firstborn over all creation. For by him all things were created: things in heaven and on earth, visible and invisible, whether thrones or powers or rulers or authorities; all things were created by him and for him. He is before all things, and in him all things hold together. And he is the head of the body, the church; he is the beginning and the firstborn from among the dead, so that in everything he might have the supremacy. For God was pleased to have all his fullness dwell in him, and through him to reconcile to himself all things, whether things on earth or things in heaven, by making peace through his blood, shed on the cross" (Colossians 1:15–20).

What does it mean that in Jesus . . .

"all things hold together"?

_____

has "supremacy" in everything?

_____

What are the implications of these divine declarations for your life?

_____

Revelation 21 and 22 picture the world to come. Take a few minutes to read these short, concluding chapters of the Bible. What strikes you about this peek into the future? What can we look forward to? How does seeing what is ahead give us hope and renewed motivation now?

_____

_____

_____

What does it tell you about the heart of our God that He is in the process of making everything new (Revelation 21:5)?

_____

_____

_____

Losing It for *Life*

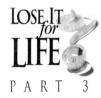

God wants us to succeed in this journey. Here's a list of questions you can use right now (and every morning before you launch out into the day), to help you remember the basics.

- Today—right now—am I surrendered to God? Even if I don't understand everything that is happening, is the attitude of my heart, "Not my will, but Thy will be done"? If not, what's keeping me from this?

- Today—right now—am I engaged and involved deeply with other Christians? Even when I feel like pulling away? Today—right now—am I participating in healthy community? If not, what's keeping me from this?

- Today—right now—am I giving trusted friends the right to hold me accountable and ask me hard questions in love? If not, what's keeping me from this?

- Today—right now—am I being honest, real, and authentic? Have a renounced a lifestyle of pretending to be what I'm not? If not, what's keeping me from this?

- Today—right now—am I working on renewing my mind—replacing old distorted and unhealthy thinking with God's truth (as revealed in His Word)? How so? What's my plan for today? If not, what's keeping me from this?

- Today—right now—am I maintaining clear boundaries to keep me from returning to sick, sinful behaviors? If not, what's keeping me from this?

- Today—right now—am I committed to forgiving others quickly; that is, keeping short accounts? If not, what's keeping me from this?

- Today—right now—am I being patient with myself when I slip, remembering God's grace and the truth that my journey is a marathon, not a sprint. (Note to self: One misstep or even 20 wrong steps will not wipe me out.) If not, what's keeping me from this?

"So don't lose a minute in building on what you've been given, complementing your basic faith with good character, spiritual understanding, alert discipline, passionate patience, reverent wonder, warm friendliness, and generous love, each dimension fitting into and developing the others. With these qualities active and growing in your lives, no grass will grow under your feet, no day will pass without its reward as you mature in your experience of our Master Jesus. Without these qualities you can't see what's right before you, oblivious that your old sinful life has been wiped off the books" (2 Peter 1:5–9, THE MESSAGE).

Dear Lord,
Grant me the
serenity to
accept things I
cannot change,
the courage to
change the
things I can,
and the
wisdom to
know the
difference.
Amen.

For Use in a Group Setting

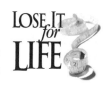

Each participant should have a *Lose It for Life* book and *Workbook*. Because the *Workbook* follows the 11 book chapters, it will work best in an 11-week format. The workbook has five lessons (days) for each chapter of the book. Each week, discuss the first lesson (Day 1) for each chapter with your group. Then make sure that everyone finishes the next four days of lessons during the week.

Preparation

To prepare for each week, participants should read the appropriate chapter in the book and then work through the corresponding "week" in the *Workbook*, being sure to answer all the questions. You, as the group leader, should do the same.

Openers

You may want to begin each session with an interesting "opener" to introduce the topic and initiate discussion. These activities should be light and easy to do. When used well, openers can be very effective. As you think through your own creative openers, here are some sample ideas:

- To begin the Week 1 session, distribute magazines and have group members find ads for diet plans or articles about losing weight. Then ask, "What are the most popular diet plans these days? Which ones have you've tried over the course of your life?"

- Week 2, show the "Red Pill" clip from *The Matrix* video or DVD.

- Week 3, have the group design a new "breakthrough" diet that focuses on the guidelines you give. For example, break into pairs and have them create a diet centered around the colors "orange and yellow"; a "left-overs only" diet; a "timed" diet (everything must be consumed within a certain time limit), and so forth. Use your imagination. Everyone will enjoy some good laughs as they hear the "diet" reported. And this will lead naturally into the topic.

After the first week, you may want to precede the opener with a brief time of personal reporting/reviewing. Ask members how they did during the week, and be sure to affirm those who completed their assignments.

Discussion

You'll notice that some of the questions in the LIFL *Workbook* are more personal than others. To avoid embarrassing anyone and keep the discussion moving, choose the more neutral questions to highlight in the group sessions. (Note: the "Losing It for Life" section of each lesson focuses on personal application.) Eventually, you will be able to get more personal, especially in Week 10, where we discuss holding each other accountable. You may even want to have group members divide into "accountability partners." *(Note: It's important to foster an environment of confidentiality within the group as they share experiences.)*

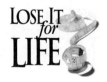

Wrap-up

The end of the lesson is the time to encourage members to continue doing the lessons and to follow through on their assignments. You may also want to end with a time of prayer, so members can pray with and for each other.

Endnotes

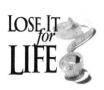

Week 1: What Do You Have to Lose?

1. Nancy Hellmich, "Obesity in America is worse than ever," *USA Today* (October 9, 2002).

Week 2: Take the Red Pill

1. Tara Parker-Pope, "The diet that works: What science tells us about weight loss," *Wall Street Journal* (April 22, 2003).

2. Ibid.

Week 4: The Doctor Is "In"

1. "Causes of obesity," Mayo clinic, *Women's Health Source,* (April 2002), Vol. 6, No. 4.

2. Retrieved on-line May 11, 2004 from http://instruct1.cit.cornell.edu/courses/ns421/BMR.html

3. Retrieved on-line May 11, 2004 from http://instruct1.cit.cornell.edu/courses/ns421/BMR.html

4. J. Hoffman, "Why does fat deposit on the thighs and hips of women and around the stomachs of men?" Scientific America.com (May 23, 2004). Retrieved on line May 23, 2004 at http://www.sciam.com/askexpert_question.cfm?articleID=000D5A77-FA90-1D89-B3B9809EC588EEDF&pageNumber=2&catID=3

5. Denise Mann, "Stress may cause fat around the midsection in lean women," article on WebMD.com (September 22, 2000). Retrieved May 23, 2004 on-line at http://my.webmd.com/content/article/28/1728_61643.htm?lastselectedguid={5FE84E90-BC77-4056-A91C-9531713CA348}

6. Robert K. Su. Posted in the Virginia Pain Clinic, Portsmouth Virginia (1985). Used with permission.

7. http://www.niddk.nih.gov/health/nutrit/pubs/health.htm#diabetes, Retrieved April 29, 2004.

8. Ibid. http://www.niddk.nih.gov/health/nutrit/pubs/health.htm#heartdisease

9. Ibid.

10. http://www.niddk.nih.gov/health/nutrit/pubs/health.htm#sleep

11. http://www.niddk.nih.gov/health/nutrit/pubs/health.htm#gallbladder

12. http://www.niddk.nih.gov/health/nutrit/pubs/health.htm#liver

Week 5: Nutrition Transformed!

1. "The society for neuroscience. Brain briefings: Sugar addiction," (October 2003). Retrieved on-line from http://web.sfn.org/content/Publications/BrainBriefings/sugar.html

2. Charles Platkin, "If you want to lose weight, you need more than a miracle food," *The Honolulu Advisor*, (November 27, 2002).

3. Lisa Davis, "Holy cow, look what makes you thin," *Reader's Digest* (July 2002), 107–111.

4. "Oreos too dangerous for our kids, suit says," *The Orange County Register,* the AP (May 13, 2003).

5. Samantha Heller, "The Hidden Killer," *Men's Health* (September 2003), 116–118.

6. Nutritional briefs in *Men's Health* (May 2003), 50.

Week 6: Move It and Lose It

1. "Fitness Fundamentals," developed by the President's Council on Physical Fitness and Sports. Retrieved on-line June 2, 2004 from http://www.hoptechno.com/book11.htm

2. J. Wilmore, "Exercise, obesity and weight control," retrieved on-line June 3, 2004 from http://www.fitness.gov/activity/activity7/obesity/obesity.html

Week 7: Coming Out (of the Eating Closet)

1. Based on questions adapted from Linda Mintle, *Breaking Free from Compulsive Overeating,* (Lake Mary, Fla: Charisma House, 2002).

Week 10: Community—the Connection Cornerstone

1. R. Stuart, "Do intimate partners help or hinder weight loss?" *Psychology Today* (Jan/Feb. 2002), 43.

THE TOTAL SOLUTION
—PHYSICAL, EMOTIONAL, SPIRITUAL—
FOR PERMANENT WEIGHT LOSS

LOSE IT *for* LIFE

STEVE ARTERBURN & DR. LINDA MINTLE

No diet, pill or surgery can give you God's tools to Lose It For Life.

But this book can.

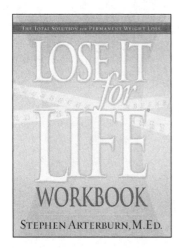

Most diet programs only tell you what to eat or how to exercise. And when you're done with them, the pounds return. *Lose It For Life* is a uniquely balanced, total solution that focuses on your mind, body and soul—and how the emotional, mental and spiritual factors affect your weight. Ultimately, this solution—developed by best-selling author and radio personality Stephen Arterburn, who lost 60 pounds 20 years ago and has kept it off—helps readers achieve what they desire most: permanent results.

Using the principles from the nationally recognized Lose It For Life Seminars, this groundbreaking book is the perfect companion to any weight-loss program—Atkins, South Beach, Weight Watchers, whatever! And it's co-authored by Dr. Linda Mintle, whose clinical work in eating disorders gives even more hope to those who have tried diet fads with disappointing results.

This book will give you the information and motivation you need to live a healthy life and to finally *Lose It For Life!*

ISBN 10: 1-59145-245-7
PRICE: $22.99 U.S.

Lose It For Life for Teens
Steve Arterburn & Ginger Garrett

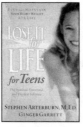

Weight is such a critical issue with teenagers. They are overwhelmed with messages that present unrealistic and unhealthy body images. *Lose It For Life for Teens* will save them a lifetime of struggles and negative self-perceptions. It will help young people:
• deal with emotional triggers for overeating
• set the right goals
• understand how to lose weight in a healthy way and keep it off
• design a customized work-out program
• realize the power, comfort and relational support God offers.

ISBN 10: 1-59145-248-1
PRICE: $12.99

Lose It For Life Workbook

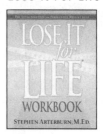

This companion workbook helps participants to better apply the program to their specific situation. It is also ideal for group study, helping facilitate meetings for those who want to encourage each other in their journey toward better physical and spiritual health.

ISBN 10: 1-59145-275-9
PRICE: $13.99 U.S.

Lose It For Life Day by Day Devotional

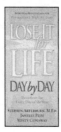

God is interested in all of our problems, but surprisingly, many Christians neglect or are reluctant to bring their struggles with weight issues to Him. *The Lose It For Life Day by Day Devotional* will help Lose It For Lifers draw daily spiritual encouragement from the One who loves us most and is interested in every aspect of our lives—even our struggles with weight.

ISBN 10: 1-59145-249-X
PRICE: $13.99 U.S.

Lose It For Life Journal Planner

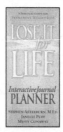

The *Lose It For Life Journal Planner* is a vital tool that will help participants plan for success and record results on their journey toward optimum health. It also includes valuable specific support for those days when temptation is hitting hardest.

ISBN 10: 1-59145-274-0
PRICE: $9.99 U.S.